Dying in the Twenty-First Century

Basic Bioethics
Arthur Caplan, editor

A complete list of the series appears at the back of the book.

Dying in the Twenty-First Century

Toward a New Ethical Framework for the Art of Dying Well

edited by Lydia S. Dugdale, MD

The MIT Press
Cambridge, Massachusetts
London, England

First MIT Press paperback edition, 2017

© 2015 Massachusetts Institute of Technology

Set in Stone by the MIT Press.

Library of Congress Cataloging-in-Publication Data

Dying in the twenty-first century : towards a new ethical framework for the art of dying well / Edited by Lydia S. Dugdale, MD.
    pages cm.   (Basic bioethics)
Includes bibliographical references and index.
ISBN 978-0-262-02912-4 (hardcover : alk. paper), 978-0-262-53459-8 (pb)
1. Death--Moral and ethical aspects. I. Dugdale, Lydia S., 1977- editor.
BJ1409.5.D95 2015
179.7   dc23
                                                                    2014046102

for Diana

Contents

Series Foreword

Glenn McGee and I developed the Basic Bioethics series and collaborated as series coeditors from 1998 to 2008. In Fall 2008 and Spring 2009 the series was reconstituted, with a new Editorial Board, under my sole editorship. I am pleased to present the forty-fifth book in the series.

The Basic Bioethics series makes innovative works in bioethics available to a broad audience and introduces seminal scholarly manuscripts, state-of-the-art reference works, and textbooks. Topics engaged include the philosophy of medicine, advancing genetics and biotechnology, end-of-life care, health and social policy, and the empirical study of biomedical life. Interdisciplinary work is encouraged.

Arthur Caplan

Acknowledgments

Many colleagues, collaborators, friends, and family members have supported this book project. I offer my sincere thanks to:

• Autumn Ridenour, for suggesting that I submit an article to the *Hastings Center Report*'s fortieth-anniversary call for papers, and the *Hastings Center Report* for printing it. An unnamed colleague read that article and encouraged me to put together a book proposal, and Daniel Callahan suggested that I submit the proposal to the MIT Press.

• Pamela Maddock and the late Allen Verhey, for reviewing the initial book proposal. Allen kindly provided me with an early draft of *The Christian Art of Dying*.

• The MIT Press, for accepting the book proposal. Clay Morgan, Philip Laughlin, and Miranda Martin graciously entertained my countless questions. Paul Bethge is an unending source of editorial wisdom.

• Patrick O'Connor, my section chief at the Yale School of Medicine, for instruction on how to navigate the uncharted waters of editing a volume.

• Mark Mercurio, Director of Yale's Program for Biomedical Ethics, for his continuous support of my scholarship.

• Thomas Duffy, who, among his numerous roles at Yale, has been my co-director of (and co-conspirator in) the Faculty Bioethics Journal Club.

• Matthew Ellman, Peter Ellis, Katherine McKenzie, and Lisa Puglisi, physician colleagues at Yale Internal Medicine Associates and sources of encouragement. I am especially grateful to Matthew for reviewing a draft of chapter 1, and to Katherine for her many literary suggestions.

• Members of our office staff, who have provided much continued cheer for this project. For the last two years, Theresa Harris has asked me at least quarterly for updates on the book's status. Christine Golden has kept me fed. I am also grateful to Jessica Kaslow, Alisa Gordon, Diana Alvarez, Elizabeth Chernes, Yvonne Augur, Laura Marshall, Blossom Linton, Orimena Givens, and Louise Wallace for their daily help in the clinic.

• My patients Diana, Geraldine, Virginia, Wilbert, and William, whose ongoing discussions with me about living and dying have been invaluable. I especially wish to thank Diana for her thoughtful review of the concluding chapter.

• The Program on Medicine and Religion at the University of Chicago. Although I started this project before I became a Faculty Scholar in the program, funding from the John Templeton Foundation enabled me to complete the book. I thank the co-directors of the Program on Medicine and Religion, Daniel Sulmasy and Farr Curlin, and my fellow scholars Michael Balboni, Amy DeBaets, John Hardt, Warren Kinghorn, Abraham Nussbaum, Aasim Padela, and Elena Salmoirago-Blotcher. I also thank Daniel Kim, Emily Chen, and Maha Ahmad for their logistical support.

• Mark Siegler of the University of Chicago, for inviting me to pursue medical ethics. I believe his precise words, some ten years ago, were "Lydia, you should do ethics." As a consequence, my career to date has been so much richer than I could have ever imagined. Mark and his wife Anna have been constant sources of encouragement professionally and personally. I am grateful to Mrs. Kay Bucksbaum and the Bucksbaum Institute for Clinical Excellence, of which Mark is the Executive Director, for supporting a special conference on the themes of this book. Many thanks also to Angela Pace-Moody and Sara Corderman of the Bucksbaum Institute for organizing the conference in masterly fashion.

• The contributors to this volume, Jeffrey Bishop, Lisa Cahill, Daniel Callahan, Farr Curlin, Michelle Harrington, John Lantos, Stephen Latham, Therese Lysaught, Autumn Ridenour, Peter Selwyn, and Daniel Sulmasy.

• My parents, siblings, and extended family, whose support has been constant.

• Eloise and Susannah, who remind me daily of the importance of living well, and Kyle, who reminds me daily of the chief end to which we live.

I   Setting the Stage for a Contemporary Art of Dying

1 Dying, a Lost Art

Lydia S. Dugdale

The outbreak of the Bubonic Plague in the fourteenth century claimed the lives of up to two-thirds of Europe's population and thrust death to the forefront of human consciousness. The Plague struck with a uniformly fatal blow, and less than a week separated early sickness from death. Few clergy survived to attend to the dying or bury the dead, and the laity lacked the expertise to perform proper burials in the custom of the Catholic Church. Conscious of the potentially eternal consequences of improper attention to dying and death, the Church responded with a call for the articulation of an *Ars moriendi*, or *art of dying*, that could guide laypersons in their preparation for death. This initiative subsequently gave birth to a body of literature that gained mass appeal, circulated widely, and shaped both religious and secular practices in the West for several hundred years.

Late in the nineteenth century, as Western societies grew increasingly concerned with the art of *living*, practices concerned with dying were largely neglected. Scientific advance came to represent progress, and death suggested failure. By the middle of the twentieth century, technology's ability to delay the moment of death fostered a "medicalized" death. Hardly an "art," medicalized dying is perhaps more aptly described as a *technique* of dying or as a *technical approach* to death. It replaced the practices and prayers of the *Ars moriendi* with procedures and protocols for the efficient management of patients in intensive care units (ICUs). Yet at certain moments in the latter half of the twentieth century, death briefly recaptured public attention, particularly during the "death and dying" movement of the 1960s and the 1970s (which followed the introduction of the intensive care unit, organ transplantation, and cardiopulmonary resuscitation) and during the emergence of AIDS in the 1980s. Both of these moments affected how particular individuals and their communities thought of dying, but neither had a lasting effect on the broader society's approach to death; that is, neither prompted a return to an *Ars moriendi*.

It therefore remains true that Americans in general are not well equipped for the experience of dying. The reasons for this are many. Perhaps most obvious among them is the fact that Americans don't see death. Increasingly, it has been relocated from the home to the institution, and technological advance has obscured the distinction between the living and the dying. I recall standing alongside the family members of patients who have been repeatedly admitted to and discharged from an ICU. As a physician, I may be fully aware that this time the patient will not survive. But to family members, the patient looks much the same during his or her last visit to the ICU as during the first. The sedated, mechanically ventilated body appears much the same whether transiently ill or dead.

Beyond this "obscuring factor" of technology, other things contribute to the lack of preparedness for death. Many people struggle to accept death's reality—even physicians, who have firsthand experience with it. But many patients, and even some physicians, pledge an unwavering faith in technology's capacities: "With technology, all things are possible." But technology doesn't enable us to face our fears or confront what unsettles us about death.

The rise of a pluralist culture has further confounded the tasks of preparing for death. Western society lacks consensus on broader existential questions: on the purpose of life, on the significance of death, and on the possibility of an afterlife. In contrast to the religious substructure of the *Ars moriendi*, the secularization of Western culture, and of biomedicine in particular, has marginalized the role of religion. Until the middle of the nineteenth century, the doctor might have ceded his position to the priest when healing proved impossible, but now physicians control the life-sustaining technology that delays the moment of death. And even though hospital-based chaplains have a greater presence now than a few decades ago, it is ultimately the doctors who have supplanted the priests at the deathbed. Yet physicians remain notoriously ill-equipped to address issues of death and dying with their patients. And religious institutions—themselves not exempt from the secularizing forces of society—have shirked their responsibilities to help prepare their parishioners for the afterlife in which they profess to believe.

Although the field of bioethics has, since its earliest days, debated end-of-life issues, it has offered no definitive guidance to the broader public.

The challenge, then, is to outline a framework for aiding a diverse population to prepare for death. In order for such a framework to support the retrieval of an art of dying, it must both meet the needs of a plural society and prove relatively easy to adopt. In the chapters that follow, bioethicists take up this challenge.

Ethics, Not Theology

Before attempting to assess the necessary framework for a contemporary art of dying, it is worth asking why the framing should be ethical, even *bio*ethical, in nature. If the original *Ars moriendi* emerged from within the Catholic Church, one might ask whether one should not then look to religion to provide a new framework for preparing for death. Is not death, in the view of many, a transcendent experience? Indeed, as the palliative care physician and ethicist Farr Curlin explains in chapter 4, most patients *want* their doctors to ask them about their spiritual or religious needs, particularly as they approach death.

The language of medical science, however, is not the language of religion. Curlin has noted elsewhere that more than half of physicians in the United States claim that their religious beliefs influence their practice of medicine, and that those religious characteristics are diverse, with varied implications for practice.[1] Though individual clinicians may feel equipped to address the spiritual concerns of dying patients, many more would, no doubt, shy away from it—and perhaps with good reason.

Furthermore, the discourse of contemporary religion lacks consensus. In the fifteenth century, the vast majority of Western Europe's population could look without hesitation to the Catholic Church for answers to existential questions. No such religious authority exists today in American society. The bioethicist Stephen Latham notes in chapter 3 that approaches to dying have varied significantly across time periods, places, and cultures. Latham draws on the work of Joanne Lynn, another bioethicist, who observes that Americans typically die in one of three ways: either they maintain good function despite a known illness until a sudden decline leads to death, or they suffer from a chronic condition characterized by periodic exacerbations and remissions, or they retain generally healthy bodies but deteriorate cognitively. All three patterns of dying involve significant reliance upon health care. Thus, preparing patients for death falls to the health care system. As a result, the language of medical science has come to be spoken universally, in contrast to the language of religion.

Contemporary bioethics, then, is the common tongue for moral discernment, for conflict resolution, and for descriptions of normative practices within biomedicine. In pursuit of these aims, bioethics has a tradition of drawing on philosophy, theology, law, medicine, politics, the life sciences, and other disciplines. Although discomfort with the language of religion has led to the marginalization of theology within bioethical discourse, Lisa Cahill has argued, "it is more appropriate to construe theological contributions as overlapping and coinciding with philosophical ones, than to see secular, philosophical bioethics and religious, theological bioethics as two distinct or even competing entities. ... Public bioethical discourse (or public policy discourse) is actually a meeting ground of the diverse moral traditions that make up our society."[2] In chapter 5 of this book, the ethicist-theologian M. Therese Lysaught casts doubt on the ability of bioethics to deliver the depth of content necessary for meaningful moral deliberations about death. Lysaught suggests that bioethics as currently practiced is insufficient for the task of helping individuals to die well and that the methodology of bioethics should include virtue ethics. One might argue instead that what is required in order to be able to articulate a contemporary art of dying is a robust bioethics that doesn't shy away from the richness of the philosophical and theological traditions, but rather engages them.

Preparation for Death

As a preface to the articulation of a latter-day *Ars moriendi*, I will outline the evolution of Western approaches to death, focusing on five historical moments: the Bubonic Plague, the American Civil War, the advent of intensive care and life support, the death and dying movement, and the AIDS crisis. Though these moments may seem disparate, each moment had an effect on societal approaches to death.

The Bubonic Plague
As I have already noted, in 1347, the Bubonic Plague (also called the "Black Death," because infected flesh turned black) claimed nearly two-thirds of Europe's population, and typically less than a week passed between the first sign of illness and death. According to historical records, the death count

rose so quickly that the living could scarcely manage to attend to the dying or conduct proper burials. Since priesthood conferred no special immunity to the Plague, a pressing need arose for a mechanism that would enable parishioners to prepare for death in the absence of clergy.

The Catholic Church, then Western Europe's leading religious authority, responded to the perceived need by issuing texts, collectively known as the *Ars moriendi*, to guide the laity in preparation for death. These books emphasize that a Christian can prepare for a good death by leading a repentant and righteous life. They argue that the dying faithful should not fear death, since God is in control of every moment, including death itself. The texts warn against temptations to unbelief, despair, impatience, pride, and avarice, and lead the dying through a series of questions for reaffirming belief and receiving consolation. The *Ars moriendi* texts also prescribe specific practices and prayers that might be performed by attendants on behalf of the dying—activities that would, in turn, encourage them to prepare for their own deaths.

The books were quickly translated and circulated throughout Europe. Over the course of the next several centuries, as the Black Death continued to strike—in Seville in 1647, in London in 1665, in Vienna in 1679, in Marseille in 1720—the *Ars moriendi* literature was adopted, modified, and redefined by non-Catholic religions, always with a view to preparing the faithful to die well. Such books remained in wide circulation, including in the United States, until the end of the nineteenth century.

The American Civil War

Americans of the Civil War generation were certainly acquainted with the art of dying. Jeremy Taylor's 1651 revision of the *Ars moriendi*, titled *The Rule and Exercise of Holy Dying*, had established the genre within Protestantism, which dominated nineteenth-century America's religious landscape. But by the 1860s concepts of a "good death" had moved beyond the domain of religion and into mainstream culture, promoted in stories, poetry, and music. Elements of a good death had become, as the historian Drew Faust notes, "as much a part of respectable … behavior and expectation in North and South as they were the product or emblem of any particular religious affiliation."[3]

But the Civil War forced a radical rethinking of death. The war was, in effect, a plague, affecting nearly every household. An estimated 620,000 soldiers died, a number exceeding deaths in the Spanish-American War, the two world wars, and the Korean War combined; some historians contend that even this is a gross underestimate.[4] Although before the war Americans had been accustomed to high infant mortality, those who survived childhood were expected to live at least into middle age.

But it was not simply the numbers that compelled Americans to rethink death. "Death's significance for the Civil War generation," Faust writes, "arose as well from its violation of prevailing assumptions about life's proper end—about who should die, when and where, and under what circumstances."[5] Young men snatched from the fullness of life gave themselves in service to the cause of country. No longer solely a matter of God receiving his faithful into eternal glory, death became patriotic; sacrifice connoted citizenship and honor. Soldiers would routinely ask that their families be informed of their courage in battle should they not survive. According to Faust, "dying bravely and manfully became an important part of dying well."[6]

The Civil War also changed the context in which death was experienced. Nineteenth-century deathbed practices stemmed from the *Ars moriendi*. Death was a domestic affair in which loved ones ministered to and received direction from the dying. Around the deathbed family members sought reconciliation and made peace. War, however, offered no guarantee that soldiers could die at home; often they died far away, in the company of strangers or even enemies. Families were unable to comfort their dying loved ones, to record their last words, or to reconcile differences.

In addition, the magnitude of the destruction wrought by the war forced the United States to restructure its national commitments toward dead soldiers and their families. At the start of the war, the armies had no formal process for registering the graves of dead soldiers, providing for decent burials, or notifying next of kin, nor were there national cemeteries. By the war's end, five national cemeteries had been established, and when it was practicable the Union dead were gathered from around Southern battlefields and re-interred in burial grounds maintained by the federal government. When bodies were moved to centrally managed cemeteries, death was distanced from and symbolically transplanted out of the communities of the deceased. Death became a national commitment, and national commitments, in turn, shaped death.

Thus, the Civil War forced death out of the community—with its traditions, rituals, and religions—and into the public sphere, in which death and the associated practices were recontextualized. Death came under the domain of the state and the hospital, and the deathbed ritual began to lose its appeal. After the war, churches began to deemphasize the concept of dying well and to promote instead the notion of living well. And within an increasingly secularized society, the advances of medical science offered new glimpses of an immortality achievable on Earth.

The Advent of the ICU

Society was thus prepared for the promises offered by cardiopulmonary resuscitation and intensive care: promises of an indefinitely prolonged life. And such new technology furthered the distancing of death from an *Ars moriendi* model in two ways: by permanently removing death from the purview of the community; and by transferring power over life and death to the doctor.

Though after the Civil War the United States returned briefly to familiar habits of dying at home, that didn't last long. In 1908, according to the Bureau of Health, 14 percent of all deaths in the US occurred in institutions, most of them hospitals. But by 1914 the percentage had jumped to 25.[7] In the early 1930s, as reports emerged about doctors' experiences of caring for and resuscitating critically ill patients in recovery rooms (which functioned as "the first ICUs"), the hospital gained increasing importance.[8] By the middle of the twentieth century, half of all the Americans who died did so in a hospital, and in the 1990s the percentage was closer to 80.[9] Although by 2009 only about a quarter of deaths occurred in hospitals, another 42 percent of Medicare beneficiaries died in hospices; nearly one-third of them had been there for three days or less.[10] Death in an institution, shrouded from view, remains the norm today; the community rarely bears witness to the process of dying or participates in the rituals associated with preparing for death. In chapter 5, M. Therese Lysaught expounds on this new geography of death.

At this point one might object that the hospital cannot force the dying to discard traditional community practices at the door. While this may be true in theory, two distinct cultures cannot coexist without the dominant affecting the weaker. And the culture of medicine, as the physician and philosopher Jeffrey Bishop explains, has developed its own belief systems, to which the dying are subjected when they elect institutional care: "Medicine believes that it can respond with technologies and techniques to the stranger without violation. ... Whether Jewish or Christian or Muslim or Hindu or agnostic, we are all one under medicine's assessments and operationalized definitions. ... Through its techniques, medicine dilutes difference into the sameness of the assessments."[11] Bishop argues that, as the culture of medicine seeks to systematize the care of the dying, it *disembodies* patients, cutting them off from "the histories, capacities, projects, and purposes into which they have been initiated by a community." Whereas respect for community practices might become, in the ICU, a matter of assigning the appropriate social worker or chaplain, a question of the sort that the *Ars moriendi* sought to address would by met by no such consultant.

The introduction of cardiopulmonary resuscitation and intensive care also furthered the secularization of death practices through a power transfer from the clergy to the doctors. Before the middle of the nineteenth century, the doctor would give way to the patient's priest as death drew nigh; but with the advent of new technology, the physician became the keeper of the keys to everlasting life. Bishop contends that the ICU "has created the illusion of individual immortality. ... It is a different quest from the one pursued by religion, for it is no longer a search for a life after death, but rather an attempt to maintain material life and function indefinitely."[12] Such a contention might, to some doctors, appear hyperbolic. "We care for our patients with vexing uncertainty," they might say. "Courses of illness can wax and wane for years, and as physicians we are constantly discussing with patients the risks and benefits of treatment, the chances of recovery, and the goals of care. It is not simply a matter of keeping the patient alive at all costs." But although Bishop would recognize that the practice of medicine is extremely complex, his intention is to show that the overall thrust of medicine is toward action; and there exists within medicine no greater locus of action than the ICU. By contrast, when it comes to death, the patient would be better served by an *art* of dying than by the *action* of applied technology. In chapter 4, Farr Curlin further considers how a technological approach has become the default pathway for dying.

One can readily follow the implications of this paradigm shift. As doctors became the gatekeepers of death-delaying technology, the line between life and death became increasingly blurred. Ordinary people, who previously had little difficulty discerning when a person had died, now relied upon experts to determine whether a patient was good-and-alive, barely alive, or dead-but-appearing-alive. Patients entered the black box of the

ICU, received various interventions, and exited, often in a state of restored health. When they left the black box in a state approaching death, death often came without warning, leaving little time for preparation. Uncertainty over death's imminence was exacerbated by doctors' unwillingness to confront death or relay bad news, or by their notorious inaccuracy at prognosticating.[13] Thus, a hope in technology's salvific powers, combined with an ecclesiastical emphasis on an art of living well, all immersed in medicine's own culture of maintaining the functions of the animal-machine, provided the necessary set of conditions to isolate the process of dying from a religious context. Indeed, dying *lost* its process and became instead a decision about whether to disconnect machines; withdrawal of life support became its own kind of deathbed ritual.

The Death and Dying Movement

In his 1955 essay "The Pornography of Death," the anthropologist Geoffrey Gorer reacted against what I have labeled the "black box" of the ICU. In a new kind of prudery, death, which had once been a welcomed subject of discussion even for children, became "unmentionable." It came to be considered "as disgusting as the natural processes of birth and copulation were a century ago."[14] According to Gorer, such mid-century "prudery" stood in stark contrast to the deathbed scene so common to Victorian and Edwardian prose, "one of the relatively few experiences that an author could be fairly sure would have been shared by the vast majority of his readers." In the middle of the twentieth century, as also happened with other social taboos, death became fascinating, even titillating.[15]

It was against this backdrop that the death and dying movement gathered momentum in the late 1960s and the 1970s. Medical practitioners began to recognize the absurdities of the life-at-all-costs, black-box model of care for the dying. Both within the realm of medicine and in society at large, there was a renewal of interest in speaking of death openly and plainly. Many in the profession of medicine responded to calls for such conversations.[16] In 1967, Cicely Saunders launched the hospice movement in the United Kingdom by opening Saint Christopher's Hospice. The psychiatrist Elisabeth Kübler-Ross fueled the conversation with her popular 1969 book *On Death and Dying*. Instead of calling society back to an art of dying, however, Kübler-Ross proposed a scientific description of the stages of psychological reactions to death. According to Bishop,

As a product of a member of the medical establishment, her work was central to the movement of medicine from the pursuit of technological mastery of death to the pursuit of psychological mastery of death—to owning death, to accepting it. She succeeded where other, more scientifically, psychiatrically, and psychologically rigorous accounts that had appeared before hers could not have succeeded. However, it is also clear that she gave the five stages of dying/grief a scientific veneer, with the result that the five stages could be heard and accepted by those who would master death technologically.[17]

Bishop goes on to show how Kübler-Ross's work led to an explosion of grief-assessment tools, reinforcing medicine's technological mastery of death with the supplemental pursuit of a psychological mastery—all ostensibly quite distant from an *art* of dying.

Others, however, see Kübler-Ross's work as helping to inspire an art of dying through the establishment of the hospice movement in the United States. In 1968, Dean Florence Wald of the Yale School of Nursing took a sabbatical to work with Cicely Saunders at Saint Christopher's Hospice. In 1972, Elisabeth Kübler-Ross testified on the subject of "death with dignity" before the US Senate Special Committee on Aging; two years later, Florence Wald founded America's first hospice.[18] And yet, although the death and dying movement and the hospice movement have done much to improve contemporary care of the dying, both fall short of reinvigorating an *art* of dying, a point Farr Curlin addresses more fully in chapter 4. Perhaps a crisis beyond the control of biomedicine, such the emergence of a new and devastating infectious disease, could revive the *Ars moriendi*.

The AIDS Crisis

In the 1980s, AIDS—not unlike the Plague—stripped away youthful illusions that life would never end. And for a brief period, AIDS changed the medical establishment's approach to death. One doctor recalls that in the early days of AIDS the medical team at his New York hospital made rounds with a rabbi, a pastor, and a funeral director.[19] AIDS forced medicine to recognize that preparation for death was an important aspect of caring for patients. It is worth noting, however, that because those who were affected by AIDS were largely members of marginalized populations, and because of medicine's quick response to the disease in the form of pharmacotherapy, AIDS didn't have a lasting effect on how society at large approached death. Peter Selwyn takes up this subject in chapter 10.

Toward a New Ethical Framework for the Art of Dying Well

The evolution of practices surrounding death can thus be traced through a series of steps: from a nearly universal art, to a matter of national interest, to an expert-driven implementation of technology, to an object of scientific and therapeutic mastery. This overview is limited and omits much, but it clearly reveals that the *Ars moriendi* tradition, which spanned more than 500 years, has gone the way of its earlier practitioners.

The goal of this book is to begin to articulate a bioethical framework for a contemporary art of dying; but before we can even attempt such a task, we must recategorize death from unmentionable to mentionable, and even to anticipated. In chapter 2, Jeffrey Bishop takes up the subject of human finitude and demonstrates how finitude threatens both the dying and their doctors. Our finitude both brings into focus the things we value most and takes them from us. It demands of us, Bishop argues, a kind of humility before the complexity that characterizes the human being, a humility that seems a prerequisite for the recovery of an *Ars moriendi*.

In chapter 3, building on Bishop's chapter, Stephen Latham addresses the question of whether plural approaches to death are merely relative. He begins with the notion that, over time and across cultures, humans have conceived of many different types of death as "good." He then analyzes this plurality of types of death by drawing from the German philosopher Nicolai Hartmann's work on the hierarchy of values. The achievement of high values—such as universal love or artistic beauty—is praiseworthy. It is a great wrong to deprive a person of strong values such as those of health and life. By giving consideration to strong values but reaching for high values—even in dying—Latham shows that a good death is not simply relative.

In chapter 4, Farr Curlin takes up Latham's argument that not all deaths can be considered "good." Curlin explores current practices of hospice and palliative medicine and shows how they both recover an art of dying and undermine the spirit of the *Ars moriendi*. Curlin warns that hospice and palliative medicine, as a professionalized form of caring, has adopted some practices that don't necessarily allow for the achievement of higher values in dying—values that, as Latham shows, are necessary for the articulation of a new art of dying. Rather, Curlin suggests that hospice and palliative medicine is best practiced within medicine and under the constraints of that profession; despite a more limited role, it is within the context of medicine and its associated *telos* that hospice and palliative medicine can best help patients engage in the tasks of dying well.

The chapters in part II explore the substance of the *Ars moriendi*—rituals and practices, spiritual preparation, and the role of community. In chapter 5, M. Therese Lysaught argues that, whereas rituals and practices had played important roles in the art of dying from the Middle Ages until the early twentieth century, today they are ambiguous concepts on unsteady footing within secular biomedicine. Society has lost the rituals and practices that helped to guide patients and their communities through the dying process. Lysaught turns hesitantly toward bioethics for a solution. She draws on earlier work by Daniel Callahan, whose vision for a new art of dying turns on a person's character. Lysaught shows how "the formal, procedural logic embraced so passionately" by present-day bioethics cannot offer a robust solution without undergoing substantial changes to its own framework. All is not lost, however, and Lysaught leaves the reader with some practical steps for working toward an art of dying.

In chapter 6, Michelle Harrington and Daniel Sulmasy interweave philosophy, theology, and medicine in an exploration of the role of spiritual preparation in a contemporary art of dying. Building on Lysaught's observation that the rituals and practices of the *Ars moriendi* are meant largely for spiritual preparation for death, they address the aims of the patient autonomy movement to take control of dying and death. Through a narrative account of the life of Saint Francis of Assisi, they show that there is a freedom to be gained in choosing how to live in such a way that we may die well. The repercussions of death itself, they contend, might produce the greatest freedom.

The *Ars moriendi*, as developed over several hundred years, was practiced within the context of community. In chapter 7, the ethicist-theologians Autumn Ridenour and Lisa Cahill build on this notion as they address the role of community in the articulation of a contemporary art of dying. They question whether conventional interpretations of patient autonomy best serve the dying patient, and argue instead for Kant's notion of relational autonomy, which, in their view, corrects overly individualistic conceptions of autonomy. They show how current bioethical and philosophical views of personhood both clash with and support their call for a relational autonomy, and they conclude with practical ways in which patients, their communities, and health care professionals can collaborate to promote improved care of the dying.

The chapters in part III address special cases at the deathbed. In chapter 8, the ethicist and pediatrician John Lantos takes up the subject of the deaths of children. Attempting to make sense of the deep suffering and "radical uncertainty" that accompany such deaths, he appeals to both narrative and empirical studies. Lantos shows that how we think about critically ill children and how we care for them and their parents are important to an art of dying. Care of dying children remains an important representation of society's response to the most desperate suffering.

In chapter 9, the ethicist Daniel Callahan addresses special concerns at the opposite end of the spectrum. He invites the reader into a discussion of grief and of Alzheimer's dementia, of the moral problems facing individual caretakers, and of the broader question of intergenerational responsibility of children to care for their parents. Callahan makes use of personal narrative to provide practical guidelines for the use of life-sustaining treatment for advanced dementia. His conclusions, like so many in this volume, are limited and cautiously optimistic, and he underscores themes articulated earlier by Ridenour and Cahill pertaining to the role of community in continuing to meet the needs of the dying.

In chapter 10, Peter Selwyn, a front-line "AIDS doctor," revisits the bedsides of his dying patients, recounting the lessons learned from the early years of the disease, when no treatments were available and caregivers could do little more than stand with their patients in humble solidarity. Advances in drug therapies, however, have radically changed the nature of care for AIDS patients, and have threatened the unmediated human connection between patient and caregiver. Selwyn's comparison of early and current approaches to care of patients suffering from AIDS offers insight to all who may be tempted to hide from their own anxieties about life and death behind a thin partition of machines, drugs, and statistics.

In the concluding chapter, I collect the themes that emerge from the preceding chapters and show how together they might contribute to the rediscovery of an art of dying. I respond to the concerns raised by Lysaught and, after reconsidering whether bioethics is in fact suited to the task, conclude that only a very robust bioethics could foster both the contemplation of finitude and the cultivation of community that would be necessary for a present-day *Ars moriendi*. Returning to the rich complexities of finitude and community, I outline the obstacles that impede progress. I conclude by identifying the areas that remain to be explored, recognizing that the contours of this exploration must themselves continue to shift as the needs of dying generations change.

Acknowledgments

This chapter builds on the content of my paper "Death without God: Examining the Secularization of Death," presented at Inaugural National Conference on Medicine and Religion at the University of Chicago in 2012. Parts of the *Ars moriendi* section appeared in a substantially different form in "The Art of Dying Well," *Hastings Center Report* 40 (2010): 22–24.

Notes

1. Farr A. Curlin et al., "Religious Characteristics of U.S. Physicians: A National Survey," *Journal of General Internal Medicine* 20 (2005): 629–634.

2. Lisa Cahill, "Can Theology Have a Role in 'Public' Bioethical Discourse?" *Hastings Center Report* (1990): 10–11.

3. Drew Gilpin Faust, *This Republic of Suffering: Death and the American Civil War* (Vintage, 2008), 7.

4. Faust, *Republic of Suffering*, xi, 273n2.

5. Ibid., xii.

6. Ibid., 25.

7. Robert V. Wells, *Facing the "King of Terrors": Death and Society in an American Community* (Cambridge University Press, 2000), 195.

8. Jeffrey P. Bishop, *The Anticipatory Corpse: Medicine, Power, and the Care of the Dying* (University of Notre Dame Press, 2011), 112.

9. Sherwin B. Nuland, *How We Die: Reflections on Life's Final Chapter* (Vintage, 1993), 255.

10. Joan M. Teno et al., "Change in End-of-Life Care for Medicare Beneficiaries: Site of Death, Place of Care, and Health Care Transitions in 2000, 2005, and 2009," *Journal of the American Medical Association* 309 (2013): 470–477.

11. Bishop, *Anticipatory Corpse*, 307–308.

12. Ibid., 110.

13. Natalie C. Momen and Stephen I. G. Barclay, "Addressing 'the Elephant on the Table': Barriers to End of Life Care Conversations in Heart Failure," *Current Opinion in Supportive and Palliative Care* 5 (2011): 312–316; Karen M. Gutierrez, "Prognostic Communication of Critical Care Nurses and Physicians at End of Life," *Dimensions of Critical Care Nursing* 31 (2012): 170–182.

14. Geoffrey Gorer, "The Pornography of Death," *Encounter* (1955): 50–51.

15. Whereas Gorer penned his essay in the pre-dawn of the so-called death and dying movement, Allen Verhey, in *The Christian Art of Dying* (Eerdmans, 2011), directly tied the "pornography of death" to an increase in popular culture's fascination with death.

16. Herman Feifel, ed., *The Meaning of Death* (McGraw-Hill, 1959).

17. Bishop, *Anticipatory Corpse*, 238.

18. "History of Hospice Care," National Hospice and Palliative Care Organization (http://www.nhpco.org/history-hospice-care).

19. Gerald Friedland, conversation with author, February 4, 2011.

2 Finitude

Jeffrey P. Bishop

Any attempt to reinvigorate an *Ars moriendi* in the twenty-first century first requires the acknowledgment and acceptance of human finitude. One cannot talk of preparing for death without accepting that death is a personal and real inevitability. By way of a narrative, I will describe human finitude in its epistemological, scientific, and existential senses, showing how both patients and doctors are necessarily subject to it. Yet, I also claim that grace is possible even when we suffer at the hand of finitude.

In contrast to the gods, human finitude governs meaning; finitude seems to be both destructive of human meaning and productive of it. A number of years ago, I was reminded of this paradox. I was the weekend general internist on call when a 29-year-old woman, whom I will call Elaine, was admitted to the hospital by the neurology department.

Four years earlier, Elaine had presented to an emergency department after a seizure. She was 32 weeks pregnant, and she and her husband Jim had been out shopping for the baby's nursery. A CT scan of Elaine's head had shown an astrocytoma, a type of brain tumor. The name of the tumor is, in part, descriptive of how it looks, because it spreads throughout the substance of the brain with little "star"-like arms moving in every direction. Her tumor was staged as a grade III astrocytoma. Elaine decided to delay her treatment until after delivery. At 36 weeks, she gave birth to a healthy boy, who was named Jacob. Shortly after delivery, she underwent brain surgery and then radiation. After the treatment course, she was slightly more emotionally labile and had lost some of her inhibitions, but she was alive and able to care for her son.

A few weeks before I met Elaine, a head scan showed a recurrence of the astrocytoma. This finding was to be expected; grade III astrocytomas nearly always recur. Her neuro-oncologist decided to place her on a high dose of dexamethasone (a steroid that reduces inflammation and swelling) in addition to chemotherapy; she tolerated this treatment pretty well. Then, three days before I met her, she developed diarrhea, fever, and light-headedness. Her blood pressure was low, and she had a very low white blood cell count (WBC): 2.0. Taken together, her symptoms (diarrhea, fever, and light-headedness) and signs (low blood pressure and low WBC) suggested an infectious diarrhea. The physicians in the emergency department sent urine and stool samples for culture and discharged Elaine. In my opinion, they should have admitted her that day. Two days later, she called her neuro-oncologist, who sent her to the hospital again; this time, she had dangerously low blood pressure and WBC count, low sodium, high potassium, and significant kidney impairment. The neuro-oncologist called me in to see her, because she was gravely ill.

When I saw Elaine, she had a wild-eyed look—a look I had seen only a few times. Most people are lethargic, or not quite with it, when they are dying. A few are bright-eyed and able to answer questions, but their answers are a bit off. Elaine was just that way: bright-eyed, edgy, not quite right, but still conversant, almost vibrant, but dying nonetheless.

Elaine's heart was racing, her blood pressure was low, and she had profound electrolyte and acid-base abnormalities in her blood. She was breathing too fast. I took blood cultures, administered intravenous fluids and antibiotics, and gave her a dose of hydrocortisone to treat her adrenal problems. She was critically ill, probably in septic shock, and in need of immediate intervention if she was going to survive. I could tell that she knew she was dying (patients often know these things) and the strong face, the wild-eyed look, was in part an attempt to reassure loved ones that everything was going to be fine. Despite the fluids and the hydrocortisone, her blood pressure didn't improve and her blood became more acidic. Not only did she need a breathing tube because of her acidemia and her respiratory failure; she also needed it to help increase her oxygenation. Before I intubated her, I asked Jim to bring Jacob into the intensive care unit so that Elaine could see him for what would be the last time. She held him, kissing his cheeks and forehead. When Jim left the room with Jacob, Elaine was coherent enough to recognize the gravity of her circumstances.

Our finitude threatens all that we value, and the fact of our finitude brings into relief what we value most. That seemed obvious to Elaine, even in her state of shock. This paradox—the fact that our finitude both takes meaning and value away from us and tells us what we find meaningful and valuable—is at the heart of the human condition. In fact, in ancient societies—societies founded on myths different from late-modern Western myths—the immortals were fickle precisely because they were not limited by a finite nature. The ancient gods were petty and childish; they were willing to do all manner of things to settle a score with a fellow immortal, often at the great expense of mortal humans. But it was the fact that they didn't die that made the gods so fickle and capricious. In order for the gods to know what was valuable, they would have to be mortal. Immortality doesn't give infinite value; it would seem that only mortality does that.

Yet for us mortals it is a hard thing to admit of limitation, precisely because to do so would threaten all that we value. Our finite nature is the source of our culture. We are driven, because of our finitude, to build things that outlive us, to build a reputation that persists beyond our death, to leave a legacy behind. And we cling to medicine in our desire to avoid death, in our attempts to live a long and healthful life, in our aim to hold onto all that we value. Whereas culture is built to outlive us mere mortals, medicine—also a product of culture—is designed to stave off finitude. We practitioners of medicine are so good at technical mastery of the failing mechanisms of the body because we have, as a culture, placed medicine as one of the most important institutions in Western society. We build culture and we build medicine in order to escape the sting of death and finitude. So our finitude tells us what is important about living and dying; and medicine works to alleviate that finitude because we modern Westerners want to keep all that is important to us.

Our limited and frail bodies—the source of our finitude—are the focus of medical science and medical technology. Yet, as we desperately turn to medicine to sustain our frail and limited bodies, medical knowledge also meets its limits. That is to say, we turn to medicine to attenuate our finitude so that we can continue to enjoy the values and meanings of our lives, but even medicine is finite.

The Limits of Knowing

I placed a breathing tube in Elaine's airway and gave her pressors to enhance her blood pressure, hoping to improve blood flow to her vital organs. The fluids and the hydrocortisone didn't have the intended results. Her blood pressure didn't go up, even after I gave her the pressors. I was puzzled. Physiologically, she had low blood pressure as a result of severe septic shock combined with adrenal insufficiency. In theory, she was dehydrated as a result of the diarrhea and the massive dilation of the blood vessels caused by sepsis syndrome. She had what doctors call a "capillary leak": fluid from inside her blood vessels seeped out into her tissues. Fluids should have helped, hydrocortisone should have helped, and pressors should have helped. They did not.

Thinking I may have been wrong about Elaine's physiological situation, I called for a cardiology consult. Fortunately, the consultant was the very best physiologist of all of our cardiologists. He was also a character: ironic, cynical, confrontational, a smoker. We called him Swinging Bob. I was glad he was on call. Bob suggested that I insert a Swan-Ganz catheter through a large vein into Elaine's heart in order to measure the pressures in the heart and in the pulmonary vessels. I did that, but afterward I was even more puzzled; her numbers suggested a form of shock due to heart trouble, not to infection.

When Bob arrived, the echocardiogram showed that Elaine's heart wasn't pumping normally and that fluid was backing up into her lungs. In other words, instead of septic shock, she appeared to have cardiogenic shock. Bob suggested that we lower the dose of the dopamine pressor and try adding dobutamine, a medication that helps with heart failure. We hoped that Elaine's heart would start pumping more effectively, and it did. But her blood pressure didn't improve. It was as though the laws of physiology were upside down. I turned to Bob and asked "What do we do?" Bob looked at me and said, in his usual colorful manner, "Jeff, we're fucked! I don't think we can save her."

Now, every doctor who reads this will think that Bob and I had made some sort of error. The rules of physiology don't behave this way. Either the patient had septic shock complicated by adrenal insufficiency or she had left ventricular failure and cardiogenic shock. In reality, she probably had some elements of both—severe septic shock with toxin-mediated left ventricular dysfunction. In fact, Elaine's physiology precisely illustrates what the philosophers Samuel Gorovitz and Alasdair MacIntyre call "necessary fallibility."[1]

Years ago, Gorovitz and MacIntyre described error in science and how we typically think about error in medicine. In the natural sciences there are two forms of error. The first is error of ignorance—scientific knowledge hasn't yet progressed far enough to have answered the questions at hand. The second form of error pertains to is the individual scientist—and refers to an error of willfulness or error of negligence. But Gorovitz and MacIntyre went further, saying that there is yet another form of error found only in the applied sciences: *necessary error.*

There is a wide gap between our scientific knowledge—which is founded on the law-like generalizations of the natural sciences—and the particular patient who sits before me. We can never know whether our general knowledge about patients with septic shock is true of any particular patient. For example, with our general knowledge that 75 percent of patients respond to a therapy, we can never know whether a particular patient will respond, or to what degree, or what extraneous factors will change the patient's response. This may be attributable to many factors, such as the patient's genetic makeup or the patient's particular history (perhaps the patient would have been responsive under normal physiological circumstances, but not under the new physiological environment). Gorovitz and MacIntyre summarized this point with great clarity:

Precisely because our understanding and expectations of particulars cannot be fully spelled out merely in terms of lawlike generalizations and initial conditions, the best possible judgment may always turn out to be erroneous, and erroneous not merely because our science has not yet progressed far enough or because the scientist has been either willful or negligent, but because of the necessary fallibility of our knowledge of particulars.[2]

Gorovitz and MacIntyre's necessary fallibility is merely a statement about the finitude of knowledge. And even when the state of basic science advances to near complete knowledge, the overall complexity of any particular situation and the overlapping particulars that contribute to the whole physiological picture of a patient will mean that we cannot ultimately know or control what is happening to a patient such as Elaine. Inevitably, we medical doctors are bound to butt up against the finite nature of our knowledge and the behavior of the particulars that are so important to the particular patient who sits before us.

In the applied sciences, we must deal in particulars. Thus, our necessarily fallible knowing is always merely a hypothesis about the expected result of the application of general knowledge to the particular. Whereas a nuclear physicist doesn't need to know which particular particle or quantum of energy he or she is looking at, a physician is concerned specifically with a particular patient, a particular body's history and environment, and a particular disease. Gorovitz and MacIntyre illustrate the problem of particularity by reference to hurricanes. Though all hurricanes operate on the same universal laws of physics, it is difficult to predict the landfall, the wind speed, or the rainfall of any particular hurricane because of the complex environments that interact in its development. A storm, like a human being, can never be merely the sum total of all the chemical and physical processes involved. There are too many other contingent conditions that bear upon the creation of a storm or a response to an illness. Laws of physics that are bounded by the initial and boundary conditions might exist in the laboratory, but seldom are these known beforehand in a natural environment. The particular contingent history of a particular patient will have an unpredictable effect on the behavior of that patient's body and physiology. In Elaine's case, her diarrhea, her overall septic shock, with massive dilation of the blood vessels, the leakage of protein into the tissue outside the vessels, and her kidney failure, in combination with her adrenal problems and the impairment of the functioning of her heart muscle, made it very difficult to know precisely what should have been done for her.

Knowledge of particulars is made even more difficult by the fact that we must take the teleological element of particulars into consideration. That is, although it doesn't make sense to refer to the flourishing of atoms, it does make sense to refer to the flourishing of particular human bodies. Flourishing adds a very important dimension to our understanding of the nature of human bodies. Whereas a natural scientist must abstract from notions of flourishing in order to say what is absolutely true about subatomic particles, a meteorologist or a physician cannot do that, for he must know whether a particular storm or a particular patient is flourishing or beginning to fail. In this sense, the teleological elements of a storm and a patient are parallel. But whereas a failing storm is no longer flourishing, human flourishing is possible even as the body is failing. It is specifically in the minutes, days, and years of the body's failure that meaning—and so flourishing of another immeasurable sort—can be found. There is, then, a kind of excess that is possible for human bodies; the sign of the excess is that meaning is produced. Thus, for human bodies in their particularity, a teleological element involves not only the biological assessment of the body but also the teleological element that goes beyond the body. It isn't just that finitude threatens to take it all away, and thus meaning is produced. Grace, gratuity, and excess are possible even in a failing body; it is out of the failing body that meaning and value are produced. If a physician can't fully account for the particularities of the flourishing or failing body, surely he or she can't account for the particularities of the flourishing and/or failing that is still productive of a meaning that goes beyond the body.

Frailty, Dependency, and Death

After Bob and I recognized the gravity of Elaine's condition and the reality of our inability to explain its cause or to treat it, I told Elaine's husband Jim that her condition seemed to be worsening. Elaine's blood pressure was erratic, her urine output was falling, she remained acidemic, and we were having difficulty oxygenating her. By then, many of Elaine's friends and family members had arrived: her parents, a sister and a brother, friends from college, a high-school friend, Jim's parents. They consoled one another, held Elaine's hand, and expressed their love for her. Elaine's nurse and I entered the room periodically to answer questions and to check on her. The nurse and I even found ourselves consoling each other. We humans are able to overcome aspects of our finitude through the care of others. We are born unable to manage our own survival and would surely die without the family into which we have been born. We are perhaps the most dependent of animals, requiring circles of family members, friends, neighbors, communities, and countries to secure stability in the face of our finitude. Jacob was losing his mother, but had his father and his grandparents. Elaine's parents were losing their daughter, and would help to support Jim in raising Jacob. Our dependencies are reorganized when our final finitude manifests.

On one of my visits into the room, Jim pointed to one of the pressors and asked "What is that medicine doing?" After I explained, he asked "Is there any point in it?" I said "Well, I don't know. It doesn't seem to be helping." He asked "Then should we turn it off?" I said "I suppose we could." We did, and Elaine's blood pressure dropped some and stabilized at the lower level. Over the next hour, Jim asked about the purpose of other medications and we decided together whether each was worth continuing. Eventually, Elaine was on minimal doses of the pressors, the antibiotics, the sedatives, and the IV fluids. Her urine output diminished to nothing, her systolic blood pressure was in the 70s, and her heart rate was in the 140s—things that any clinician would recognize as indicating that she was close to death. I asked Jim if he wanted me to reinstitute any of the treatments, but he didn't. He said something to the effect that he didn't think Elaine would want to be put through all this and be kept alive by machines, especially since the cancer had returned. He said that she knew she was going to die, and that he was happy that her last conscious memory was of their son. And she was surrounded by her friends and family members, the best that any of us can hope for when our bodies fail.

Later I asked Jim if he wanted me to take Elaine off the ventilator. He said Yes. The nurse, the respiratory therapist, and I disconnected the mechanical ventilator and removed the breathing tube. As the nurse cleaned Elaine's face and made her more comfortable, I charted the decision to remove Elaine from the ventilator. We invited the family into the room and began to dial down the remaining pressors. Elaine's systolic blood pressure began to fall slowly, from the 70s into the 60s, the 50s, and the 40s. Her heart rate initially jumped, but then gradually began to decrease. Her breathing slowed from 28 breaths per minute to the teens, then gradually decreased to zero. Her heart rate dropped into the 20s, and then she flat-lined on the monitor. In contrast to the wild-eyed woman who had presented just 15 hours earlier, the woman in the bed was serene; she appeared comforted by those who had surrounded her, those upon whom she had depended the most, those whom she had loved the most, and those who loved her the most.

Unanswered and Unanswerable Questions

A few hours after Elaine's death, her blood cultures returned growing several different bacteria, suggesting that she had a massive infection, probably related to diarrhea. I had chosen a broad-spectrum antibiotic that would have covered this type of bacterial sepsis, but it hadn't been enough. Elaine's family requested that her body be sent for autopsy so that we could figure out what had happened.

A few weeks later, I received the results from the autopsy. The report was amazing. Elaine had had terrible colitis (infection of the colon), probably because of the high doses of steroids she had been given to treat her tumor. The steroids would have diminished her body's immune response to the infection, which of course meant that the infection had spread through her entire system. In other words, she had become super-infected with multiple organisms that had spread from her colon into her bloodstream, which had resulted in overwhelming sepsis.

But there was one other result in the autopsy report that turned my stomach. The autopsy report for the brain said "No sign of recurrent astrocytoma." There were no signs of the recurrence of her tumor at all. The tumor had not recurred. She hadn't needed the round of dexamethasone and chemotherapy.

How had the neuroimaging shown a recurrence? There was a clear difference between the penultimate CT and the one that showed the growth in the supposed tumor. Or was it that the scar had changed? Scar tissue doesn't grow, but something had happened to suggest that the tumor had recurred. Now, surely the imaging techniques weren't as good as they are today, but even those few years ago I was shocked that such a costly error could be made. Did the neuro-oncologist err? Should he have insisted on other tests to confirm the recurrence? Was he too aggressive with the dexamethasone? He reasoned statistically that Elaine should have been treated; and statistically he should have been correct. Statistically, the new finding on Elaine's neuro-imaging should have been tumor recurrence. Statistically, treatment with the chemotherapeutic agent and dexamethasone should have been safe for her. But statistically there will always be patients for whom our knowledge fails.

What about me—did my knowledge fail me too? Did I stop too soon? "Knowing" that the astrocytoma had recurred made me more willing to stop aggressive therapy. If I had known the tumor had not recurred, I wouldn't have been so quick to turn the pressors off or to remove the ventilator. I may have given Elaine a few days to see whether she could rebound from the illness. Did all the goodbyes, all the friends and family members, and her goodbye to her son predispose me to give up too quickly? Was the complexity of her illness and the long road to recovery, if even possible, seen as too much to overcome with the supposed brain tumor? I don't know, but these questions haunt me even today.

Ripples of Finitude

Each level of chaos and each ripple of Elaine's bodily finitude joined the ripples of our finite knowledge to create a wave of destruction for Elaine.

The failures in her body (the astrocytoma, the infection enabled by dexamethasone, the combined septic and cardiogenic shock), in conjunction with the failures in our knowledge and the failures of our therapies, surely resulted in her death. And she lost so much that was of value to her. Her family lost so much of what was of value to them; Jacob would not know his mother.

The fact of our finitude shapes what we see, and what we think we see. Did I see a dying woman, because of her physiology? Or did I see a dying woman because of the astrocytoma, which wasn't there? The fact of our finitude shapes how we think about and value what we see—the meaning and purpose of our life, what we value most, who we would want to see and with whom we would want to reconcile if we are at death's door. The flux of life—the coming into being and the passing away of things—allows that which we value most to come into relief.

Still, it is hard to think of our finitude, our death. Sure, we can see a dead body, as it presents itself as an object. Yet in our culture most people see only a few dead bodies in their lifetime. For the most part, we don't see the dead, nor do we suffer with them as they are dying. All the suffering and the dying seems to take place in a hospital, hidden from our view, under the purview of professionals. In my father's day, as late as the 1950s, it wasn't uncommon for a brother or an uncle or a grandparent to die at home surrounded by friends, family members, and children. In that way, the end of a life could be seen, could be experienced, but only in the third person. It wasn't uncommon for the body of a dead person to be laid out in the home for viewing; friends and family members would gather around and tell stories about the loved one who, as they put it, had "gone on to his reward." These practices have gone the way of small towns and small subsistence farms. With the rise of medical technology and our ability very effectively to treat any number of ailments that would have killed a person years ago, dying at home is rare. In fact, even after the rise of hospice care, the vast majority of deaths occur in hospitals. Sherwin Nuland's book *How We Die* was in part a kind of medical response to the fact that death has been removed from our cultural sight.[3] Few of us have seen actual deaths. Nuland's book, then, acts to present death and finitude as an object of inquiry, something we still experience in the third person. Some anonymous third person dies in Nuland's book. His book is really about how *they* die. Not how *we* die.

It is hard to think of *my* finitude, *my* death, because *my* death, *my* ending is not something about which *I* will be able to think. Thus, when I say
"It is hard to think of death" I don't mean merely that it is culturally hard
to think of death. G. W. F. Hegel said that death is a concept for which we
have no image or representation.[4] In Hegel's theory of knowledge, concepts
were empty containers for which the mind had to have a concrete representation. Thinking of *my* death—death in the first person—is impossible.
For when *I* die, that by which and in which and through which I know dies.
In effect, there is no conscious awareness in my death, so I literally cannot
think my own death. Heidegger puts it a different way. Where time can be
experienced but not represented existentially, death can be represented in
the other, but cannot itself be experienced.[5]

There is a way of telling this story of finitude in such a way as to suggest
that religions were born or created by humankind so that we could think
about death. If I am thinking of my death before I am dead, consciousness
persists. Consciousness persists while I'm thinking about death, even if I
can't really think of my ending. Life persists if I am thinking of my death.
For some, this persistence of consciousness as I think about death gave rise
to beliefs about life after death. Others have claimed that this is the birth of
idealism, which suggests that the ideas persist even when things pass away.[6]
My mind projects itself out beyond my time; my thinking posits itself as
existing beyond my death, because there is no way to think about death
without doing so. But then it is not my death.

Judaism gets past this problem of idealism, but not by positing a life after
death. It does so in its understanding of history and of the destiny of the people of Israel. Christianity gets past this problem of idealism and any notion
of life after death in a different way. It does so by appeal to its doctrine of the
resurrection of the body, which is not the same as life after death.

Early in the *Negative Dialectics*, Theodor Adorno states that objects "do
not go into their concepts without leaving a remainder."[7] I take Adorno
to mean that things have a kind of integrity that resists all our knowing,
or rather that things exceed our knowing even when we know them well.
Though that is certainly true for things—including bodies and persons—
that are at the apex of their flourishing, it is also true of bodies and persons
as they are failing. There is always more that can be said about things, and
there is a kind of hope in that which exceeds our knowing. In fact, there is
more that can be said about human thriving even in the face of the failing

body. Thus, in a paradoxical way, it is also from this excess—even excess in the failing body—that value is taken. It is as much from the hope of what might be as it is from the loss of what was that our value and our meaning are born. That is the reality of human bodies, and it is this reality that exceeds our knowing of bodies even as they fail. Thus, the excess that is flourishing even transforms the decaying body. In other words, there is more than mere finitude that animates the values that we place on life, for there is always hope that more is possible from bodies and from persons than even our bodies can sustain.

In the face of finitude—in the face of death—we certainly want more knowledge. But there is a way in which more knowledge will not help us. Things and our knowing of things never match up, for things are moving both as they flourish and as they fail. Flourishing and failing bodies always exceed our knowing of them. Knowledge is fleeting. What is needed, then, for existential meaning and purpose is not a better understanding of *how we die*, as Nuland suggested. Nor is it better mastery of the dying body, as is suggested by medicine's never-ending quest to sustain human life. What is needed in the face of finitude is a kind of humility before that which must remain enigmatic for us mortals. What is needed is a kind of hope that Elaine's life had meaning and purpose that exceeded her dying, even as her dying body exceeded medical and scientific comprehension.

Finitude, which threatens all that is valuable to us mortals, also animates the production of medical technology. The result has been a shift in the cultural frame through which we envision and imagine death. But whatever the cultural frame, finitude and death escape our knowing and our control. In fact, fear of death remains latent in medical technology, and medicine allows us to avoid the reality of finitude. The only satisfactory answer to finitude, it seems to me, is a kind of humility before the complexity of human being and human value—a humility that the *Ars moriendi* seems to invite. And because of the great excess that is the flourishing body—both in its living and in its dying—there is always hope that something infinite, something that exceeds our knowing, awaits us.

Acknowledgments

I thank Rachelle Barina, Devan Stahl, Emily Trancik, and Cyndy Bishop for reviewing earlier versions of the manuscript.

Notes

1. Samuel Gorovitz and Alasdair MacIntyre, "Toward a Theory of Medical Fallibility," *Journal of Medicine and Philosophy* 1 (1976): 62.

2. Ibid.

3. Sherwin B. Nuland, *How We Die: Reflections on Life's Final Chapter* (Random House, 1994).

4. G. W. F Hegel, *Phenomenology of Spirit*, tr. Arnold V. Miller (Oxford University Press, 1977), 308.

5. Martin Heidegger, *Kant and the Problem of Metaphysics* (Indiana University Press, 1962), 108; Heidegger, *Being and Time*, tr. Joan Stambaugh (State University of New York Press, 1996), 20–21.

6. Robert W. Jenson, *On Thinking the Human: Resolutions to Difficult Notions* (Eerdmans, 2003), 3–4.

7. Theodor Adorno, *Negative Dialectics*, tr. E. B. Ashton (Seabury, 1973), 5.

3 Pluralism and the "Good" Death

Stephen R. Latham

To his friend Cotton Mather, the Puritan physician and Harvard president Leonard Hoar confessed that he had long prayed, if God were willing to grant him such a bounty, to be permitted to die of "a consumptive and lingering distemper."[1] Hoar had written a tract on death, and, like most serious Puritans, had thought about the matter deeply. Not for him a sudden and painless death; he wanted a death that gave him time: time to wean himself from this vain world, time to set his soul aright, time to exhort his family members to learn from his death about the shortness of their own days.

Over the millennia we humans have reckoned many very different kinds of death "good." Hoar's desires seem very different from those of the modern Jain who stops eating when death approaches in order to demonstrate the superiority of his soul over the petty needs and wants of his body, the Viking who desired to die of battle wounds, the archaic Greek to whom the possession of a beautiful youthful body at death was preferable to the possession of one that had been marred by long aging, the Japanese for whom suicide was honorable, and the medieval Catholic for whom suicide was an appalling sin.

Anyone who thinks about the variety of approaches to death may be led to the relativist conclusion that goodness in death is purely in the eye of the beholder. But we need not make this move from variety to wholesale relativism. In this chapter I shall offer a very modest, but I think plausible, theory that explains why many different ways of dying may appropriately be characterized as good, but that leaves room for the judgment that some ways of dying are definitively bad. I will then use the theory to show why a very common contemporary way of dying—the medicalized way—is very often not good. I will conclude the chapter with some suggestions about how we might improve our practices of death.

My proposed "theory" of the good death is hardly a theory at all; it is perhaps only a conceptual vocabulary, and a small one at that, with which to discuss our preferences about death. I will be relying, here, on a modest and wholly unoriginal notion from value theory—specifically from the work of Nicolai Hartmann, a leading German philosopher of the first half of the twentieth century. Hartmann's idea has to do with hierarchy among values. For Hartmann, not all values are equally valuable, or valuable for the same reasons.[2] Hartmann drew a distinction between "high" values and "strong" values, and claimed that height and strength of values were in inverse proportion to one another.

Laying Groundwork

Before discussing the height/strength distinction, I wish to emphasize how very little of Hartmann's—or of anyone's—value theory I mean to import. I intend my use of the distinction to entail a minimum of metaethical commitments about value. For the distinction to be useful, we need not accept value realism (the view that values are objectively "out there" to be discovered and described, in the way that cows and computers are). We need not even have a particularly well-worked-out definition of values.

Provisionally, let us assume that values are qualities of persons, things, or states of affairs that it is appropriate for persons to value. We appropriately value virtues in persons, strength and speed in horses, reliability in engines, and transparency in governance. (The business about "being appropriate" is meant only to signal that something doesn't become a value just because someone, somewhere, happens once to value it. Whether what makes an instance of valuing "appropriate" is some objective assessment of the thing valued, or some culture-bound intersubjective judgment, or the product of an individual's reflective equilibrium, or some other process I leave undecided.) "Value" here is closely related to the judgment of goodness; according to Elizabeth Anderson, "to judge that something is good is to say that it is properly valued. And to judge that it is bad is to judge that it is properly disvalued."[3]

With this vague idea of "value" in place, we need accept only some fairly straightforward theses about the place of values in our moral lives. For example:

• Each of us has and pursues various values. Different cultures place heavier emphases on different values: some cultures have been more martial, some more sensitive to honor, and some more consumerist than others. And the values their members have pursued have varied with those characteristics. Within different cultures, individuals' care for and pursuit of values also differs, though some cultures are more uniform than others.

• Many values have corresponding dis-values. Honor and dishonor, transparency and secrecy, stability and instability, are obvious examples. Sometimes dis-values are harder to name: health as "the silence of the body" has multiple dis-values, including disability and pain. In general we have stronger aversions to certain dis-values than we have attractions to their corresponding values: we dread pain, but we don't particularly appreciate or honor its absence; similarly with fear and anxiety.[4]

• Various major spheres of human activity—political, scientific, artistic, romantic, economic, religious, and so on—are associated with various values. The association is difficult to articulate, but it goes something like this: Values guide activity within any sphere insofar as people within that sphere are working to instantiate, through their work, the values associated with that sphere. Politicians aim at justice, interest satisfaction, equality, or pragmatic workability. Artists aim, perhaps, at truth, expressivity, self-revelation, sublimity, or "interest." Scientists aim at non-falsifiability, predictability, and perhaps at elegance. This variation means that values that may be important in one sphere of life can be very unimportant in another. One example is efficiency, which might be valued highly in economic activity but less highly in religious or artistic activities. Another is fame, which is notoriously valued in the political sphere but may be of little value in the religious. Justice is a central value of politics, but has a much smaller place in science.

• Values can conflict, not only across spheres of activity (as when religious values of purity clash with political values of tolerance) but also within them (as when the value of equality conflicts with that of liberty in politics). I make no particular claims about what spheres of activity there are—whether they are finite in number, how continuous they are with one another, and so on. To continue, I need only the idea that different sorts of human activities are associated with different values and the idea that these values can conflict.

I take all these claims to be fairly non-controversial, not least because I mean them only to track ordinary language about value, without digging any more deeply toward underlying metaethical commitments. If I have excited controversy, my preferred response would be to pare down these claims in order to avoid it—to dodge questions rather than to answer them.

Values High, Strong, Low, and Weak

A value is "high," on Hartmann's view, if its achievement (what I am calling its instantiation through activity) merits great praise. A value is "strong" if one's being deprived of it is a great wrong. (One is deprived of a value if its corresponding dis-value is instantiated through activity, or if the value's instantiation is destroyed.) Stability is a strong value in politics; a regime that lacks stability does its citizens great harm. On the other hand, for a regime to be stable is not particularly to its credit. Stability is a strong value, but not a particularly high one. It is basic, in the sense that only a stable regime can hope to become great; but it is also low. "Low" here is no insult—we are talking, after all, about values. The correct metaphor here might be architectural: the strongest and most basic building blocks are low, and they are the condition of the possibility of reaching great heights with less strong building materials.

High values are those whose fulfillment confers greatest merit—universal love, for example, or artistic beauty. "A sin against the lower values," Hartmann writes, "is blameworthy, is dishonorable, excites indignation, their fulfillment reaches only the level of propriety, without rising higher. The violation, on the other hand, of the higher values, has indeed the character of a moral defect, but has nothing degrading in it, while the realization of these values can have something exalting in it, something liberating, indeed inspiring."[5] Hartmann cites as an example heroism—a high value that warrants admiration, even though a lack of it doesn't arouse contempt or indignation. Trustworthiness, on the other hand, is a very strong but low (and basic) moral value. Merely being trustworthy is no great moral achievement; lack of trustworthiness warrants contempt.

Life and health are, for most of us, the quintessential strong values. A person who deprives another of life, or who injures someone's health, has greatly wronged the other person. But no one deserves much praise merely for being alive and healthy. Being alive and healthy is merely the baseline from which a person can hope to achieve higher things.

Note, however, that although low, strong values tend to be simpler than higher, weaker ones, and although our higher values tend to depend upon and be constructed upon the achievement (consolidation?) of the lower ones, low and high values can come into conflict. One can deliberately sacrifice one's health for one's art, and one can choose to die for the sake of justice. In such cases, the achievement of higher values comes at the expense of lower, stronger ones.

Note, too, that not all cultures have agreed about the status of life as a value. There are today some people who might argue that life, far from being a baseline from which higher values might be achieved, is itself the highest value; the idea that life might ever be sacrificed for the sake of something "higher" seems appalling to them, the product of deeply mistaken ideology. And of course there are others (Buddhists, for example) for whom the value of life (and particularly the idea of life as a strong foundation for all other values) is deeply questionable.

Values in and of Occupations

Most occupations stand in distinct relation to two different sets of values: the values an occupation seeks to instantiate through its work and the values necessary for its practice. Mechanical engineering, for example, may aim at several values: cost effectiveness, reliability, elegance, ease of use. Those who teach and learn about the practice of engineering must learn to recognize and appreciate those values. But the values they pursue in their own calling as engineers are different. It may be important for an engineer to value the history of her field, but she need not embody any such value in her work. Indeed, the values instantiated through a practice may conflict with those necessary to conduct the practice well; consider the notorious case of the aggressive, secretive, loyal attorney who operates within a system designed to produce dispassionate, transparent, neutral rules of conduct.

The aims of medicine are, for the most part, strong and low values: medical practice is designed to restore people to health, to reduce and avoid suffering, and to stave off preventable death. It has not been an aim of medical practice to make patients courageous, magnanimous, sensitive; the aim thus far has been to restore them to their own baselines of physical and mental health, in order to free them to pursue higher values on their own. On the other hand, there are many high values necessary to the practice of medicine, and more that are exhibited in the practice of medicine at its best. One's doctor must be more than alive and healthy; she must be learned, prudent, articulate, possessed of practical wisdom, and sometimes courageous.

Values and Death

A person's death is bad insofar as it violates that person's strong values; a death is good insofar as it enables high values to be instantiated or affirmed.

Life and health and absence of suffering are all strong values; a death is bad insofar as it violates these values. Religious values, family values, or aesthetic values are high; a death that permits such high values to be instantiated or affirmed is, insofar as it does so, good.

Most deaths, of course, involve a certain amount of suffering, anxiety, or boredom; all involve loss of life. So no death is completely "not bad." A certain amount of badness can be redeemed, however, by the chance to achieve high values. Think of a person dying of cancer who turns down pain medication in order to be clear-headed when communicating with family members. The higher values affirmed in those final communications overwhelm the violations of lower, stronger values, and make the death, on the whole, good. Even an extreme case of suffering—the suffering caused by being eaten alive by a lion, for example—might be redeemed by the achievement of a high value; thus, it can be argued that martyrs have good deaths.

We can see that this fairly simple schema can very quickly explain the views, among various different societies over time, that very different sorts of death are "good." The higher values celebrated in different societies have of course been different; a Viking's good martial death is very different from the good romantic death of Young Werther. But we can also see that this variety doesn't imply a pure relativism about the goodness or badness of death. A death that involves violation of low values (suffering, anxiety, loss of life) that isn't redeemed by some compensating achievement of higher value (patriotism, courage, religious fidelity, family love) is, everywhere and always, a bad death. A death that minimizes violation of low values and permits the achievement of higher values is a good death. Closer cases are those in which the achievement of higher values is purchased at the expense of violation of strong, low values—except perhaps in some extreme cases of martyrdom or martial glory, in which one's very willingness to suffer deep violation of the strongest values is taken, by sufferer and observer alike, as the primary evidence of one's having attained the highest.

Let us consider a few recent deaths and see how this distinction between high and strong values leads us to think about them.

• Mrs. M. was diagnosed with advanced and already untreatable cancer, and was hospitalized very shortly thereafter. When it became plain that she would die within a matter of days, she informed her six children (all of them grown, and some with families of their own) and gathered them, from various parts of the country, to her bedside. On what she anticipated would be the last day of her life, she spent a little bit of private time with each of them, giving them advice, apologizing for past misunderstandings, and assuring them of her love; then she lay quietly with all of them gathered around her. Strangely, in the last hour of her life, she received a "get well" phone call from an acquaintance who clearly didn't understand the severity of her illness; she mustered the energy to handle the call with grace, accepting the poorly informed caller's chipper well-wishing and thanking her for the call, never letting on about the severity of her situation. Her children, witnessing the call, felt proud of their mother's kind treatment of the caller. When the call was ended, she made a little joke and then, gathering all of her children's hands together in her own, charged them all with taking care of one another. A few minutes later she fell into a final sleep from which she didn't awaken. She was 70 years old.

• Mrs. V., in her late 60s, initially attributed her new difficulty with walking to a wintertime fall from which she seemed not to have fully recovered. After a few months, though, came the devastating news of a diagnosis of amyotrophic lateral sclerosis (ALS). In the ensuing years, she gradually lost more and more mobility. First she couldn't walk. Then she lost her ability to play the piano, and eventually, after several years, the ability to eat on her own. She suffered from repeated episodes of depression as her world became smaller and smaller. But she threw herself into advocacy for ALS patients, working on fundraising and joining a lawsuit aimed at securing better physical-therapy benefits. Eventually she was communicating only by means of a typing machine that could sense which letter she was looking at when she blinked. In early November of her seventh year with ALS, she instructed her husband to phone her children with the news that she would shortly stop her tube feeding because she was no longer enjoying life. But Thanksgiving came and went with no sign of any change. Gradually her children guessed that she was delaying her now-desired death in order that it not mar the holiday season. Sure enough, she ceased her tube-feeding in early January and died, peacefully and at home, within days. She left a carefully composed goodbye letter to each of her children, her children-in-law, and her grandchildren.

• Professor N. was in her early sixties. She was a much-respected professor—one of the few women of her generation in her field—and was enjoying seeing her former graduate students emerge as leading scholars. She led a fiercely intellectual life, and showed no signs of slowing down. She was writing actively, teaching a full schedule, taking on new students, and engaging in academic debate with verve, energy, and an intimidating amount of historical knowledge. She was happily married with grown and successful children. One weekend day, while gardening in her yard, she simply keeled over and died of what appeared to be a massive stroke.

• At 80, Mr. S. was in his seventh year of an Alzheimer's diagnosis. The early, mildest phases of his dementia had been toughest on him, because he could sense that he was slipping and feared what might happen to him as he lost more and more capacity. But after a couple of years he was no longer aware of his dementia. For several years he lived from day to day, cared for by his wife. He would hover around her, awaiting instruction about what to do next. Even as he lost more and more of his old self, his wife continued to value his sheer physical presence. She relied on him to help her around the house with physical tasks she couldn't do on her own, and she found comfort in having the man she loved physically by her side, even as caring for him became more and more burdensome. Eventually he developed a temper, and, particularly in the early evenings, started becoming physically aggressive in a way that his old self would have found shameful. When he became too difficult for his wife to handle, she moved him, with considerable regret, into a nearby nursing home. She visited him there every day, taking home his laundry in the evenings. He looked forward to her visits, and leapt up enthusiastically to greet her whenever she arrived, even though he was no longer certain whether she was his wife or his sister. Only a few months after his entry into the home, on the morning of their 55th wedding anniversary, as he stood up from sitting on his bedside in order to accompany her into the nursing home's day room, he collapsed with a massive heart attack. He was dead by the time his wife's cries for help brought nursing staff into the room—a matter of seconds. She was holding his hand when he died, and she kissed him before his body was removed from the room. She never had to make any difficult decisions about complicated end-of-life medical interventions for him. She never had to decide whether or when to let him go.

Mrs. M.'s death from widely metastatic cancer is of the sort already briefly discussed. She certainly suffered at the end of her life, and thus had several of her strong values violated. But she suffered minimally and only very near the end of life. She never lost capacity, and she had the time to arrange for the kind of deathbed scene she desired. She managed, both through her communication with her children and through her sensitive treatment of her ill-informed caller, to affirm a number of her highest values. This affirmation seems to me to be important enough for her death to be judged "good."

Mrs. V.'s death from ALS seems also to be good on the whole. Her suffering was perhaps more profound, and certainly longer lasting, than Mrs. M.'s; she knew that she was suffering from a fatal illness for years in advance of her death, and she spent years immobilized, whereas Mrs. M. spent only a few days in the hospital. Nonetheless, Mrs. V., too, was able to affirm many of her highest values. She was able to communicate in writing with all the members of her family, and to demonstrate by the manner and timing of her death her consideration and love for them. Her chance to arrange the timing of her death in such a way as (she perceived) would not burden her family—even though it meant that she would live through several extra physically and mentally difficult months—is an important part of what makes her death a good one.

Our evaluation of Mrs. V.'s death, though, raises a difficult question: When was her death, and how long did it last? It strikes me as implausible that her death began with the onset of her fatal illness. But there is no particular reason to believe that her death began with her own decision to die; or with her decision in January to cease receiving artificial nutrition. Which "length" of death we choose might conceivably make a difference to our evaluation of it, particularly if we conceive of ourselves as balancing a quantity of violations of strong values against a quantity of affirmations and instantiations of high values. But I don't think the conception I am advancing here—of violation of strong values by a death as redeemed by achievement of high values through it—is really such a scientistic matter of weighing. Our ideas of "importance" and "comparative importance" of values need not commit us to metaphors of weight and balancing.

The death of Professor N. seems to me to present a difficult case. She did not seem to suffer at all. She may never have been aware that she was dying. She continued with her active and satisfying life until the very moment she keeled over. From the point of view of strong values, her death was the best—or the least bad—possible. No one would say she had a "hard" or a "bad" death. And yet hers doesn't strike me as a good death, either, precisely because of the complete absence of any chance to achieve any higher values. Nothing about the manner of her death said anything about her, or permitted her to affirm anything about or to herself. Her death was shocking to others, a cutting off rather than a winding up. Indeed, it seems hardly to have been a death at all, but only a sort of perishing.

And what of Mr. S.? No one wants to become demented, though a great many Americans die after a long experience of dementia. But, as with Mrs. V., we face the question of whether we may evaluate a death separately from the experience of the illness that leads to it. When did Mr. S. begin to die? Again, my inclination is to think that the question whether someone experiences a good death should be separable from questions about the cruelty of his final illness or the quality of his last years. By the time of what I am tempted to call his death, the demented Mr. S. was subjectively happy with his life; he didn't know any better. He died suddenly, without warning, and with a minimum of suffering. His death therefore seems to resemble Professor N.'s—not hard or bad, but not "good" either, not least because by the time of his death there were very few values other than the lowest and strongest to which he was attached. On the other hand, one might argue that, through pure luck, the timing and manner of his death made it a good one—if not for him, for his wife. She was left with a strong sense of closure: it was their anniversary day; she was there to say goodbye to him; and the suddenness of his death relieved her of any burden of having to make decisions about whether to subject him to any invasive or painful or confusing medical interventions, and of any doubts as to whether she had done enough to care for him.

The example of Mr. S.'s death therefore raises at least three important questions. The first, already mentioned, has to do with our ideas about when death occurs, and in particular whether the entire experience of a fatal illness is to count as part of the death. My inclination is to think that one's death doesn't always encompass the whole of one's fatal illness or even accident; one's death, I think, ought to be understood as limited to the final stages of the dying process. But I'm not sure I'm right about that; nor am I sure how much hangs on the determination, in terms of evaluating the quality of others' deaths. Second, there is the question of whether luck—the fact that a death happens to fall on a particularly symbolic date, or happens to trigger a particular legal event, or was strikingly similar to an earlier death in the family—can affect the quality of the death. I am fairly certain that it can do so, precisely by lending to the death (accidentally, as it were) some ability to affirm or instantiate higher values. And third, there is the question of whether it is legitimate to evaluate a person's death from points of view other than the dying person's own. I would argue that it is completely legitimate, and that therefore, though Mr. S.'s death was neither good nor bad from his own point of view (it was, like Professor N.'s, a non-event for him), it was a good death from the point of view of his wife.

The Medicalized Death

Most Americans, when surveyed, say they want a death rather like Mrs. M.'s, except that they want it to take place in their homes rather than in the hospital. A large majority of Americans express a desire to die at home, surrounded by their loved ones. This implies that the death will come with some warning, allowing some time for making plans. Unfortunately, though the numbers have been slightly better in recent years, it is still the case that more than 70 percent of Americans die in hospitals or nursing homes, and a large percentage die after a disconcerting series of institutional admissions and re-admissions.[6] What has happened is that death has been medicalized, as Lydia Dugdale notes in chapter 1, and this medicalization, with its attendant concentration on preventing violations of low, strong values (and particularly on the staving off of death), is interfering with people's abilities to experience deaths that permit them to demonstrate or experience higher values—love of family, rootedness, closure, religious enlightenment, and so on.

According to the bioethicist Joanne Lynn,[7] the large majority of Americans die in one of three basic ways. Like Mrs. M., about 20 percent of Americans maintain good function despite having a known fatal illness, and experience a few weeks of rapid decline as their illnesses become overwhelming and lead to death. Cancer is the most typical cause of this sort of death pattern, though not the only one. About 25 percent suffer slow decline in physical capacities punctuated by serious exacerbations, death often coming rather suddenly. A patient who survives an episode may well go home without much worsening of his everyday limitations, but at some point efforts to rescue him fail. Chronic heart failure and emphysema are the most common causes of this pattern. And about 40 percent of Americans suffer a long-term dwindling of function, requiring years of personal care. Half of these suffer serious cognitive failure. Death often follows a physiological challenge that would merely have been a minor annoyance earlier in life—for example, pneumonia, influenza, a urinary-tract infection, or a broken bone.

The first pattern of death involves intensive medical intervention in response to the final phase of rapid decline, but once the patient's real situation is confirmed, it may actually be the pattern in which it is most possible to arrange for a good, non-medicalized death. This is because the patient is aware of her fatal condition long before the final period of decline. The second pattern encourages medicalization because its bumpy road to death often involves repeated successful rescue attempts. It is difficult to anticipate which in a series of aggressive interventions will be the one that finally fails. For that reason, the patient's death is likely to include substantial technological intervention, to be fraught with the stress and anxiety caused by medical emergencies, and to take place among strangers in a strange room where one isn't even permitted to wear one's own clothes. The third pattern, too, encourages medicalization, because the condition that eventually kills the patient is often one that medicine can generally overcome. This means that both family members and medical teams are more likely to favor intensive medical interventions than to take time to create an atmosphere conducive to a good death.

There is an important caveat to be mentioned here, however: Some patients—those who place a high value on fighting their illnesses with whatever medicine has to offer—demand a medicalized death in order to help them achieve high values such as tenacity, bravery, or heroism.

The fact remains, though, that medicine's traditional focus on low, strong values such as the prevention of death—forces the dying into the intensive care unit, an atmosphere in which it is very difficult for most of us to achieve higher values. What, if anything, can be done about this?

Redeeming Death

In order to redeem the violation of low values through the achievement of high values, it would help, first of all, for patients and their families to understand the typical death patterns mentioned above. Cancer patients and others with terminal diagnoses are capable of planning their own deaths, because they understand their fates before the most aggressive medicalization begins. But patients in slow decline, with punctuated emergency visits to the hospital, may never realize that they have entered the final phase of their lives, and therefore may never be given the opportunity to trade off some of their strong values for higher ones. Similarly, the families and medical teams of patients in long-term care may be so focused on defeating the latest bout of flu or the latest infection that it never occurs to them to anticipate death. The research of Susan Mitchell has revealed that families of Alzheimer's patients seldom are aware that most Alzheimer's patients die only a few months after admission to an institution; they fail to think of Alzheimer's as a fatal illness, and therefore they fail to plan for death.[8] Persistent attention to repeated episodes of lesser, secondary illnesses means that their loved ones often die fighting for strong values in a way that excludes their achieving higher ones. Medical teams might help patients and their families realize that at some point a combative posture against death will always fail. Home hospice is a choice that, if available, seems to strike a reasonable balance between the strong value of comfort and the higher values achievable in an environment where patients and their families feel more secure and in control.

Medical teams might also help dying patients and their families to achieve high values by encouraging them to begin recognizing the dying process early on. This need not imply any advice to acquiesce to death or to cease medical interventions. The aim is simply to give people the opportunity to prepare for death as soon as it seems to be a possibility. I know that my own father and mother would have benefitted from some discussion about his death very soon after my father's Alzheimer's diagnosis. By the time I thought to have a serious conversation with my dad about what his life meant to him and to me, he no longer had anything to say, and that is a shame. As difficult as it may be for all concerned, many patients and their families would benefit if medical teams had the foresight and the courage to tell them that, though this may not be the end, it may be the beginning of the end.

Strong values ought, of course, to be given strong consideration at the end of life. All things being equal, people should not have to suffer mentally or physically if that can be prevented; nor should they die if they can be saved. But a pain-free death, though not a bad death, is not a good death either, and delaying a death doesn't make it better or worse. The good death involves reaching for something higher and less basic than the next breath. Medical caregivers, by their training, are not expert at determining for their patients and their families what that higher thing is; but they are uniquely situated to help give them the chance to reach for it.

Notes

1. Gordon E. Geddes, *Welcome Joy: Death in Puritan New England* (UMI Research, 1981), 66.

2. Nicolai Hartmann, *Moral Values: Volume 2 of Ethics* (Transaction, 2003), 44–68. See also the discussion on Hartmann on pp. 179–184 of Aurel Kolnai, *Ethics, Value and Reality* (Transaction, 2008).

3. Elizabeth Anderson, *Values in Ethics and Economics* (Harvard University Press, 1993), 3.

4. On the comparative strength of aversion, see the following essays by Aurel Kolnai: "The Standard Modes of Aversion: Fear, Disgust and Hatred," in *On Disgust* (Carus, 2004); "Morality and Practice II: The Moral Emphasis," in *Ethics, Value, and Reality: Selected Papers of Aurel Kolnai* (Athlone, 1977).

5. Hartmann, *Moral Values*, 53.

6. Pedro Gozalo et al., "End-of-Life Transitions among Nursing Home Residents with Cognitive Issues," *New England Journal of Medicine* 365, no. 13 (2011): 1212–1221.

7. Joanne Lynn, "Living Long in Fragile Health: The New Demographics Shape End of Life Care," in *Improving End of Life Care*, ed. Bruce Jennings, Gregory E. Kaebnick, and Thomas H. Murray (Hastings Center, 2005).

8. Susan Mitchell et al., "Dying with Advanced Dementia in the Nursing Home," *Archives of Internal Medicine* 164, no. 3 (2004): 321–326.

4   Hospice and Palliative Medicine's Attempt at an Art of Dying

Farr A. Curlin

In his 1974 essay "The Indignity of 'Death with Dignity,'"[1] the theologian and ethicist Paul Ramsey writes: "A few years ago, I embraced what I characterized as the oldest morality there is ... concerning responsibility toward the dying; the acceptance of death, stopping our medical interventions for all sorts of good, human reasons, only companying with the dying in their final passage. Then suddenly it appeared that altogether too many people were agreeing with me."

As a practitioner of palliative medicine, I also have embraced the "oldest morality" to which Ramsey refers. I have concluded, moreover, that with respect to the care of most dying patients, the contemporary social institutions of hospice and palliative medicine can help health professionals and laypeople to live this morality. Yet, much as Ramsey expresses dis-ease regarding a groundswell of societal enthusiasm for a "good death," I wish to express a related dis-ease regarding a groundswell of enthusiasm for the present-day practices of hospice and palliative medicine.

Largely in reaction to and as an antidote for the excesses of technological medicine, hospice and palliative medicine (HPM) has risen to prominence as a social institution for ordering the care of patients at the end of life. Despite more than 40 years of criticism from all sides, the medicalized death (the use of life-sustaining technologies to extend life as long as is possible) remains the default for North Americans who die in health care institutions, as Lydia Dugdale suggests in chapter 1. HPM, however, provides an alternative to this unartful way of dying, and it contributes to the project of recovering the practices of the *Ars moriendi* by helping to create the conditions necessary for patients and their communities to participate in the tasks of dying well (and caring well for those who are dying).

Unfortunately, HPM is susceptible to confusing the death it has power to deliver—a death with minimal suffering and (at least the appearance of) maximal control—with the good death, with dying well. This confusion makes HPM vulnerable to temptations to do away with suffering too readily by doing away with the conditions that make both suffering and dying well possible. Dying well is, in Ramsey's terms, both "a gift and a task." To be aware of the gift and to engage in the task, patients must be conscious of themselves, which means they will be conscious both of their symptoms and of their mortal condition. Such consciousness invariably includes some degree of suffering. When practitioners of HPM too quickly sacrifice consciousness in order to end suffering, they frustrate the possibility of dying well. Moreover, when HPM usurps the roles of patients and their communities in the *Ars moriendi*, HPM thereby unwittingly undermines the social trust that makes HPM practices possible.

Many patients and their families don't trust HPM and are resistant to it. I encounter such individuals in the hospital and in the community, among people of all walks of life and social strata but particularly among ethnic minorities and members of religious communities. These individuals tell stories about loved ones who declined slowly over time, fighting the good fight with the support and companionship of their family members and friends. When HPM professionals became involved in their care, their loved ones were put on powerful drugs, became unconscious and unresponsive, and were soon dead. These stories are clearly shared within communities and powerfully shape people's perceptions of HPM, which many see as a sophisticated and seductive way of getting people to die. In fear that HPM will usurp the role of the patient and that of the community in dying well, these people choose to go without the palliation that could help the patient participate in dying well.

In this chapter I propose that HPM, in order to play its proper part in serving those who are living in the face of death and to do so without undermining the possibility of patients' dying well, should locate its practices *within* medicine and subject to medicine's traditional orientation to health. Within medicine, HPM has much to offer in preserving and restoring those aspects of health that make it possible for patients to experience care and to engage in the tasks of dying well. However, when HPM is understood as a rival form of professionalized care, whose goals of minimizing suffering and maximizing "quality of life" have no necessary relation to health, the practices of HPM come to contradict the goals of both medicine (health) and the *Ars moriendi* (dying well). That will take more explaining.

HPM's Rise to Prominence

At least since the development of the ventilator, the ethical concern most often voiced regarding end-of-life care has been how to free dying patients from the unnecessary suffering and degradation caused by the overuse of life-sustaining technologies. Patients, physicians, ethicists, theologians, the religious, and the unreligious all have decried how the default pathway for those who die in health care institutions is to use life-sustaining technology to postpone death as long as is possible.

In 1996 the American Medical Association's Council on Scientific Affairs published a report titled Good Care of the Dying Patient.[2] After noting that "most Americans have difficulty accepting death as a normal physiological process" (a statement at which Ramsey might have cringed), the report lays out usual concerns that have been voiced from all quarters for decades: "In the current system of care, many dying persons suffer needlessly, burden their families, and die isolated from family and community." As the Council's words suggest, by trapping patients in a technologically driven social apparatus that imposes undue suffering and isolates them from their communities, the default pathway poses formidable barriers to dying well (and to the recovery of any art of dying).

The conventional way to address this problem, and the only strategy the Council on Scientific Affairs identified with confidence, has been to expand and enhance hospice and palliative medicine. And so HPM has been expanded and enhanced all across American health care. Innumerable waves of outreach have exhorted and assisted patients to develop advance directives that will help them fend off unwanted life-sustaining technologies when they are mortally ill and will help to pry them free of the acute care hospital and deliver them to teams of palliating health care professionals who will support their dying at home. Meanwhile, a new clinical subspecialty for HPM has been established: palliative consultation services have been added to the standard array of clinical services available at major US hospitals, and the proportion of patients dying at home and under the care of hospice institutions has been increasing steadily.[3]

However reluctant they may have been at the outset of these developments, American physicians have come to embrace HPM as the best strategy for caring for most patients at the end of life. Colleagues and I recently completed a national study of US physicians[4] in which we found that

virtually all US physicians who had cared for dying patients in the previous year had recommended that they consider hospice care. Moreover,
more than 90 percent of physicians agreed with the statement "For most
patients, hospice provides better care at the end of life than they would
receive without hospice." This is not to say that American medicine is past
the problem of overzealous use of life-sustaining technology; the default
pathway remains. Yet HPM is now a strong rival.

How HPM Fosters Recovery of the *Ars moriendi*

As a rival to the default pathway of technological medicine, hospice and
palliative medicine does much to create the conditions that would enable
patients to participate in an *Ars moriendi*. First, HPM provides an alternative
to the default pathway. Both patients and physicians have discerned that
whatever dying well entails, surely it involves more (and less) than keeping
one's "matter in motion"[5] as long as one can, isolated from one's community and under the control of machines and a system of processes that go
on with relentless and unfeeling logic. The default pathway frustrates the
Ars moriendi by putting off preparation for death through vain promises to
extend life indefinitely. The overuse of life-sustaining technology absorbs
time, energy, attention, and resources that could be devoted to other tasks
that an art of dying might entail. For example, driving back and forth to
a hospital for countless appointments leaves less time for reconciling with
one's neighbors, and it is difficult to pray or to write letters to one's children
while retching from chemotherapy. Moreover, the default pathway isolates
patients from communities (religious communities in particular) that share
a framework of meaning thick and strong enough to guide and support the
patient in the tasks of dying. If nothing else, the growth of HPM has weak-
ened the grip of this socially established default way of dying.

HPM also creates a recognizable social space in which a patient can be
described as dying and can therefore take on the dying role. One of the
refreshing aspects of my work as a hospice physician is that in my encounters with patients the pretense of fixing the problem is gone. Everyone
involved, and the patient foremost, knows that I have no further tricks in
my bag that might displace death to a point in the distant and hazy future.
Everyone is agreed that the patient is dying, not necessarily within hours
or days, but soon and for certain. This agreement has a way of focusing

attention on how to support the patient as he or she dies. For health professionals: What can be done now to be helpful in the face of certain and imminent death? For the patient: How do I go on in the face of and in preparation for the death that I cannot avoid? For members of the patient's community: What does it mean to keep faith with and company the dying person on this final part of his or her earthly journey? For patients to engage in the task of dying well, it helps for them to know and to have those around affirm that they are dying, not merely sick. HPM creates this social space, and clears it of much of the hubbub and interference that usually accompanies technological medicine.

Moreover, by locating the social space of dying within the geographical space of the home, and by opening the geographical space of the health care institution to accommodate the presence and participation of the patient's neighbors, friends, and family members, HPM removes institutional barriers that in the default pathway of technological medicine keep members of patients' communities off balance and at arm's length. The *Ars moriendi* requires the help of one's community and focuses on relationships within that community. By locating its practices within the geographical spaces of the community, HPM helps to make the patient's family members, friends, neighbors, and clergy feel welcomed and empowered to participate in the tasks of caring for the patient as the patient engages the remaining tasks of dying well.

In the social space it creates, HPM attends to the spiritual dimensions of patients' experiences. The National Consensus Project for Quality Palliative Care identifies "spiritual, religious and existential aspects of care" as the fifth of eight "core domains" of palliative care.[6] It is not alone. From the World Health Organization[7] to the International Association for Hospice & Palliative Care[8] to the Joint Commission,[9] current notions of quality end-of-life care universally include attention to the spiritual aspects of patients' experiences.

Attending to spiritual concerns is the primary focus of the *Ars moriendi* tradition, and every evidence indicates both that spiritual concerns remain central to dying patients' experiences and that patients still put great importance on fulfilling tasks related to these concerns.[10] Michelle Harrington and Daniel Sulmasy address this subject in detail in chapter 6. Most patients today welcome and even long for their health care professionals to pay attention to their spiritual concerns, *particularly* when they are dying.[11] When health care professionals do talk to patients about their spiritual concerns, patients report being more satisfied with the care they have received.[12] Such findings suggest that today's patients experience the same human longings that gave birth to the *Ars moriendi* more than 500 years ago.[13] Whereas the default pathway crowds out and diverts attention away from these longings, HPM makes attention to spiritual concerns part of standard care.

In summary, HPM seems to invite the *Ars moriendi* and to respect the space patients need to engage in it. By providing an alternative to the default pathway, by creating a social space in which a patient can take on the dying role and locating that space within the patient's community, and by treating spiritual dimensions of dying as important and worthy of attention, HPM helps to create the conditions necessary for recovering an art of dying.

How HPM Can Undermine the *Ars moriendi*

Hospice and palliative medicine, however, can also undermine and contradict the art of dying. In the first instance, with its aspiration to attend comprehensively to patients' spiritual concerns, HPM risks usurping the roles that patient, family members, and community play in preparing for death. This is particularly true when HPM pretends to deliver, professionally packaged, a form of spiritual care that substitutes for the part that a religious community would have played at the deathbed. In other words, HPM serves the *Ars moriendi* by acknowledging and attending to patients' spiritual concerns and by respecting the space needed for patients do to the spiritual work involved in dying well; and HPM usurps the *Ars moriendi* when it pretends to offer a content-full and professionalized way of managing those concerns. This hubris has been described thoroughly by Jeffrey Bishop elsewhere.[14]

More to the present point, in its efforts to relieve suffering, HPM sometimes removes the conditions that are necessary for patients to participate in an art of dying. The medications that relieve symptoms have side effects. Narcotics, tranquilizers, and anti-psychotics can be very useful for relieving pain, anxiety, and restlessness, but they can also diminish consciousness. In the *Ars moriendi* tradition, the dying person was the director of and the lead actor in a deathbed drama. But current palliating treatments render patients passive to the process of dying and therefore incapable of participating in the dramas of their own deaths.

By diminishing consciousness, these treatments also put patients existentially out of touch with their communities and their clinicians. Within the context of an art of dying, clergy, lay counselors, family members, friends, and even physicians can keep company with and be present to the suffering patient. This practice of presence is the heart of medicine. It is expressed in the term "attending physician," indicating one who attends and makes herself present to the one who is ill. Yet a patient with diminished consciousness can't experience that presence. There can be no communication, no receptivity or response, no self-conscious communion or collaboration. This is not to say that communities and clinicians can no longer care for such patients; they can and do. Yet diminished consciousness renders a patient not only passive but also dispassionate with respect to the care received. That caregivers experience such patients to be existentially out of reach is shown when caregivers comment that the patient is "not there anymore."

How are HPM practitioners to handle this tension between relieving unwanted suffering and diminishing the conditions needed for patients to die well? They cannot strictly avoid adverse side effects of palliating treatments. In attempting to do so they would fail to relieve the symptoms that not only burden patients unduly but also prevent them from engaging in the tasks of the *Ars moriendi*. The right approach, I propose, begins with recognizing that this tension results from a conflict between sometimes irreconcilable goods: the good of relieved suffering and the good of the capacity to engage self-consciously in the tasks of dying well.

Put another way, dealing with this tension begins with recognizing that relieving suffering is not the only good at stake, and that when a patient is rendered unable to participate consciously in the activities of preparing for death he or she has suffered a loss of something valuable and has failed to achieve what Latham, in chapter 3, calls a "strong" value. Indeed, consciousness, as a strong value, makes it possible for patients to achieve other high values. HPM practitioners are often in danger of not recognizing these effects of their treatments as losses, as *adverse* side effects. Indeed, it sometimes seems as if the goal of "comfort" comes to displace all other goals, and in so doing trivializes consciousness and the patient's further participation in the dying process. Indeed, some practices, such as "palliative sedation to unconsciousness,"[15] don't merely accept diminished consciousness as a foreseen if unintended side effect; they aim intentionally to make patients unconscious and keep them so until they die.

HPM as a Part of Medicine Rather than a Rival Form of Professionalized Care

I propose that, in order to allow for an *Ars moriendi* without usurping or undermining it, hospice and palliative medicine should be understood as a set of practices internal to medicine rather than as a rival form of professionalized care. As such, it should take health as its constitutive goal, with the aim of relieving suffering just insofar as suffering is related to health.

Before making a brief case for this proposal, I concede that its plausibility depends on the premise that medicine has a rational and discernible end, namely health. In some times and in some places it was axiomatic that the end of medicine was health. Aristotle wrote "Now since there are many actions, arts, and sciences, their ends also are many; the end of the medical art is health, that of shipbuilding a vessel, that of strategy victory, that of economics wealth."[16] He took these claims as starting points for philosophical reasoning, as properly basic, as things known immediately by both the many and the wise. That is no longer true. The deep cultural shifts to which Ramsey was responding have also resulted in widespread skepticism of any claims regarding the proper ends of human identities and activities, including the ends of medicine.

Despite this widespread skepticism, I will not defend here the premise that the constitutive end of medicine is health. Rather, I will attempt to show the implications of that premise for the practices of HPM. If the end of medicine is health, then palliative medicine practiced as one branch or specialty of medicine will look different than "palliative care" practiced as a broader and alternative form of professionalized caring. Within a medicine aimed at health, HPM practitioners have a rational basis for engaging in activities that preserve and restore health and for avoiding activities that diminish health or undermine the conditions necessary for patients to entrust themselves to physicians when their health is threatened or diminished.

It may seem counterintuitive to think of HPM as aiming at health. HPM, it seems, is mobilized precisely when health can no longer be restored. Yet that way of thinking misunderstands both health and the practices of HPM. Health is a positive capacity, not merely the absence of disease. Health is the "well-working of the organism as a whole," as Leon Kass memorably put it in his 1972 essay "Regarding the End of Medicine and the Pursuit of Health."[17] Health, Kass continued, is an "activity of the body in accord with its specific excellences." The health of a squirrel, for example, is displayed in the characteristic activities of squirrels, such as burying nuts, chattering, and climbing trees. Because the characteristic activities of humans are more varied, so are their expressions of health, but such expressions include the capacities to move one's bowels, to eat and digest food without vomiting, to sit or lie or walk without wracking pain, and to stay awake and to fall asleep at the proper times.

Health is also a matter of degree. HPM cannot return a cancer patient to the state of health he had before his diagnosis, but if it helps the patient go from a state of nausea, constipation, insomnia, and wracking pain to tolerating food, moving his bowels, sleeping six hours a night, and moving around free of debilitating pain, then HPM has contributed to the patient's health.

It is just these sorts of contributions to health that make it possible for patients to engage in the *Ars moriendi*, to engage the tasks of living well in the face of death. The typical tasks of the *Ars moriendi* are not physically demanding in the usual sense. They rarely involve climbing mountains or running marathons.[18] But an art of dying does require some attention, some thought, often some communication through voice or writing, and often being present relationally to others. These tasks are made extraordinarily difficult by wracking pain, breathlessness, vomiting, constipation, insomnia, and delirium. By treating and relieving these disabling symptoms, palliative medicine helps to restore the measure of health that a patient needs in order to participate actively in the task of dying well.

Here an important distinction comes into view. It is one thing for health professionals to palliate disabling symptoms with an eye to preserving and restoring a measure of health—a measure, again, that makes it possible for the patient to participate in dying well. It is another thing for health care professionals to palliate symptoms without respect to whether doing so restores health. I propose that hospice and palliative medicine should respect this distinction, embracing the former practices of palliation and resisting the latter.

HPM practitioners, however, are tempted to elide this distinction or to regard it as having no moral significance. To understand how and why they are tempted to do so, it helps to return to the cultural dynamics to which Ramsey was responding—dynamics that have only strengthened in the ensuing decades. Ramsey observed that the modern era is characterized by "increasingly mundane, naturalistic, antihumanistic" philosophies of life, in which death can be received with sanguine acceptance, but only by denying the dignity and worth of the human individual. These naturalistic philosophies don't provide frameworks of meaning strong enough to narrate suffering, death, and loss of control as something other than meaningless burdens, much less to receive these burdens as invitations to the tasks of the *Ars moriendi*.

When the meaning is gone, the suffering remains. Without a framework in which suffering, loss of control, and even dying can be received with gratitude and can disclose to the sufferer new and worthwhile tasks, the putative goal of medicine—to preserve and restore health—seems beside the point. Health for what? If no morally significant tasks remain, it seems that the minims of health that HPM might secure are goods in some abstract sense, but they are good *for nothing*. In these naturalistic philosophies of life, the only reasonable response to unwanted suffering is to be rid of it. In this context, compassion compels those who are able to relieve the suffering of their neighbors using the tools at hand. If doing so means breaking free of the traditional constraints of medicine, so be it.

Thus, HPM has come to understand itself as a broader, more holistic, more comprehensive form of professionalized care than medicine can offer. HPM has become an alternative and a rival to medicine rather than a renewal or reform movement within it. Loosed from the constraints imposed by aiming only at health, HPM has expanded its goals. For example, the World Health Organization defines "palliative care" as "an approach that *improves the quality of life* of patients and their families facing the problems associated with life-threatening illness, through the *prevention and relief of suffering* by means of early identification and impeccable assessment and treatment of pain *and other problems, physical, psychosocial and spiritual.*"[19] Note how this formulation gives HPM a seemingly boundless scope of activity. What problems, after all, are excluded from the categories of physical, psychosocial, and spiritual? Note also that in this formulation the goal is not restoring health per se, but rather relieving suffering and improving "quality of life." These goals are to be achieved through "impeccable assessment and treatment"—concepts that resonate with the vocabulary of medicine—yet neither the suffering to be relieved nor the quality of life to be maximized is necessarily related to health.

When efforts to relieve suffering and to improve quality of life are decoupled from the goal of preserving and restoring health, HPM practitioners begin to see all forms of suffering, including existential and spiritual suffering, as conditions that call for treatment. Judgments about how and to what extent each form of suffering should be relieved become loosed from traditional medical norms of proportionality that require physicians to use clinical judgment regarding what is needed and what is fitting. Because HPM is committed to maximizing patient autonomy, and because suffering and quality of life can be assessed authoritatively only by the sufferer, HPM practitioners trade clinical judgment for the direction given by "patient preferences."

The vocabulary of "patient preferences" links together the goal of control and the goal of freedom from unwanted suffering. The American Association of Hospice and Palliative Medicine makes this link explicit: "The goal of palliative care is to prevent and relieve suffering, and to support the best possible quality of life for patients and their families, regardless of their stage of disease or the need for other therapies, *in accordance with their values and preferences.*"[20] When the activities of HPM practitioners are so closely guided by "patient preferences," it makes less sense for such practitioners to limit their palliating interventions to those they believe will restore a measure of health. Indeed, many leaders within HPM now encourage HPM professionals to relieve conditions that the patient considers "unacceptable" or "intolerable."[21] No mention is made of whether the suffering is related to health.

When patients find being alive itself intolerable, then the commitment to minimize suffering and maximize quality of life, and to do so according to patients' values, can lead HPM practitioners to aim at death itself. Here I do not refer to euthanasia or physician-assisted suicide, two practices the great majority of HPM practitioners in North America still oppose. Rather, I note a shift in emphasis: HPM speaks less about relieving disabling symptoms so that patients can live as well as is possible in the face of death than it speaks about treating unwanted symptoms so that patients can die, comfortably. To give one prominent example, the National Hospice and

Palliative Care Organization describes hospice as follows: "Hospice affirms the concept of palliative care as an intensive program that enhances comfort and promotes the quality of life for individuals and their families. When cure is no longer possible, hospice recognizes that *a peaceful and comfortable death is an essential goal of health care.*"[22]

When the goal of HPM shifts from helping patients who are dying to helping patients to die, practices that render patients unconscious or hasten their death no longer seem to be last-resort options. Indeed, such practices, including palliative sedation to unconsciousness, seem to follow ineluctably from making the relief of suffering palliative care's first principle. Note the logic: HPM exists to decrease suffering and increase quality of life according to the judgment and values of the patient. A patient is suffering and experiences poor quality of life. The patient doesn't inhabit a narrative in which the suffering has meaning. The HPM practitioner has the tools to make the suffering go away by making the condition that makes the suffering possible—consciousness—go away. Although intentionally and permanently ending consciousness contradicts the goal of preserving and restoring health, HPM is an alternative and more comprehensive form of care that is not constrained by such goals. Therefore, it is permissible and perhaps morally obligatory for the HPM practitioner to sedate the patient to unconsciousness until he dies.

Why turn back? Why circumscribe HPM practices to those that preserve and restore patients' health, particularly when doing so seems an affront to compassionate efforts to relieve suffering? To begin, boundaries help keep a practice from going astray. They guard against the temptations to which certain practices are susceptible. With respect to HPM, the health-directed aims of medicine guard against the pretense of delivering a good death and against the temptation to relieve suffering by removing capacities that display health.

By limiting a practice, boundaries also license that practice to act with energy and freedom within those limits. Consider one of the boundaries expressed in the Hippocratic Oath: "I will neither give a deadly drug to anybody if asked for it, nor will I make a suggestion to this effect." In a way, this oath functions as a sort of Ulysses contract. Physicians who care for suffering patients know that both they and their patients will at times be tempted to escape suffering by intentionally ending a patient's life. It is an understandable temptation, one that can be felt very strongly. ("Surely, doctor, you are not going to abandon me to my suffering?") In taking the Hippocratic Oath, physicians have for centuries "bound themselves to the mast" by swearing never to give a deadly drug to a patient for the purpose of ending life, no matter how much the patient implores.

Physicians do not thereby abandon patients. Rather, they establish boundaries within which patients can entrust themselves to the deadly power of physicians, and within which physicians can give themselves the necessary freedom to work aggressively to restore some small measure of health to those who are dying—especially when that measure of health is just rest and relief from wracking pain or other symptoms. Physicians can give themselves freedom because they know, and their patients know, that they will not *intentionally* hasten the death of their patients. By keeping palliation within the boundaries set by the goals of medicine (both the prescription to aim at preserving and restoring health and the proscription against intentionally diminishing the patient's health or hastening the patient's death), HPM practitioners gain a similar freedom. They are free to work aggressively to relieve the symptoms that diminish a patient's health.

The question of trust is paramount. In our plural culture, people have trusted institutional medicine in no small part because the constitutive goal of medicine—to preserve and restore health—is a goal shared broadly across diverse moral traditions and communities. Assisting patients to die is not a goal shared in the same way. How and to what extent suffering should be treated is also a subject of widespread disagreements, particularly when that suffering is not obviously related to health. Already the work of HPM is inhibited by the fact that many Americans, particularly among minorities and in some religious communities, are suspicious that HPM has unmoored itself from the constraints of the rest of medicine, moving from proportionate palliation to rationalized processes of making people dead. HPM professionals erode the public trust needed for physicians to provide appropriate palliation when those professionals too easily diminish the capacities that allow patients to engage in the tasks of dying well, when they set themselves outside the traditional constraints and goals of medicine, and when they fail to recognize and respect the value of what was once called the *Ars moriendi*. To the extent that patients distrust HPM, they will go without all of the good HPM can do to contribute to the conditions necessary for dying well.

Conclusion

When hospice and palliative medicine seeks to end rather than to mitigate suffering, it frustrates and even circumvents the possibility of dying well and prevents the achievement of the higher values discussed by Latham in the preceding chapter. This error can be avoided with a form of humility—not resignation or passivity in the face of suffering, but rather the humility that recognizes that dying well is an activity for the patient and for his or her community. HPM contributes to dying well insofar as it helps to make the activity possible (by mitigating distressing symptoms, maintaining function, locating dying within the community, providing realistic information, and reassuring presence); it subverts dying well insofar as it presumes to deliver a good death by removing the capacities that make suffering possible. By setting palliation within and under the constraints of medicine, rather than as an alternative and more expansive form of professionalized care, HPM can sustain a proper humility and can focus on a limited but very important role. Rather than usurping or undermining the *Ars moriendi*, it would serve to create the conditions needed for patients to engage in the tasks of dying well.

Notes

1. Paul Ramsey, "The Indignity of 'Death with Dignity,'" *Hastings Center Studies* 2, no. 2 (1974): 47.

2. Ronald M. Davis et al., "Good Care of the Dying Patient," *Journal of the American Medical Association* 275, no. 6 (1996): 474-478.

3. Joan M. Teno et al., "Change in End-of-Life Care for Medicare Beneficiaries: Site of Death, Place of Care, and Health Care Transitions in 2000, 2005, and 2009," *Journal of the American Medical Association* 309, no. 5 (2013): 470–477.

4. Micah T. Prochaska et al., "Physician Demographic Characteristics and Attitudes Toward End of Life Hospice Care" (in preparation).

5. Jeffrey P. Bishop, *The Anticipatory Corpse: Medicine, Power, and the Care of the Dying* (University of Notre Dame Press, 2011), 60.

6. National Consensus Project for Quality Palliative Care, "National Consensus Project Articles" (http://www.nationalconsensusproject.org/DisplayPage.aspx?Title=NCP%20Articles).

7. "Palliative care is an approach that improves the quality of life of patients and their families facing the problems associated with life-threatening illness, through the prevention and relief of suffering by means of early identification and impeccable assessment and treatment of pain and other problems, physical, psychosocial and *spiritual*." Source: "WHO Definition of Palliative Care" (http://www.who.int/cancer/palliative/definition/en); emphasis added.

8. "For patients with active, progressive, far-advanced disease, the goals of palliative care are to provide relief from pain and other physical symptoms, to maximise the quality of life, to provide psychosocial and *spiritual care*, to provide support to help the family during the patient's illness and bereavement." Source: "What Is Palliative Care?" International Association for Hospice & Palliative Care (http://hospicecare.com/about-iahpc/publications/manuals-guidelines-books/getting-started/5-what-is-palliative-care); emphasis added.

9. "Spiritual Assessment," The Joint Commission (http://www.jointcommission.org/standards_information/jcfaqdetails.aspx?StandardsFaqId=290&ProgramId=47).

10. In the Coping with Cancer study, Tracy Balboni and colleagues found that 68 percent of 343 patients in the Boston area with advanced cancer reported that their religion was very important to them, and the proportions were even higher among African American (89 percent) and Hispanic (79 percent) participants ("Religiousness and Spiritual Support Among Advanced Cancer Patients and Associations with End-of-Life Treatment Preferences and Quality of Life," *Journal of Clinical Oncology* 25, no. 5, 2007: 555–560). Further study of a subset of patients found that 78 percent said religion or spirituality had been important to their cancer experience, and 74 percent indicated that their religion or spirituality played a central role in their ability to cope with cancer (Sara R. Alcorn et al., "If God Wanted Me Yesterday, I Wouldn't Be Here Today," *Journal of Palliative Medicine* 13, no. 5, 2010: 581–588.). Harold Koenig similarly found that among 542 hospitalized patients at Duke University in Durham, North Carolina, 67 percent reported that their religion was important to their coping with illness ("Religious Attitudes and Practices of Hospitalized Medically Ill Older Adults," *International Journal of Geriatric Psychiatry* 13, no. 4, 1998: 213–224). Also in Durham, Karen Steinhauser and colleagues conducted a series of focus-group studies with people involved in end-of-life care ("In Search of a Good Death: Observations of Patients, Families, and Providers," *Annals of Internal Medicine* 132, no. 10, 2000: 825–832). One of the six components of a good death that emerged was "completion," which often involves explicitly spiritual and religious dimensions. In a follow-up study ("Factors Considered Important at the End of Life by Patients, Family, Physicians, and Other Care Providers," *Journal of the American Medical Association* 284, no. 19, 2000: 2476–2482), Steinhauser and colleagues conducted "a cross-sectional, stratified random national survey of seriously ill patients, recently bereaved family members, physicians, and other care providers." Subjects were asked to rate the importance of 44 attributes of end-of-life experience that had emerged from the previous qualitative study. Notably, 89 percent of

patients (and 65 percent of physicians) indicated that to "be at peace with God" was very important. High proportions of patients, and significant though usually smaller proportions of physicians, also indicated that the following spiritually related tasks were very important: to pray (85 percent of patients, 55 percent of physicians), to feel that one's life is complete (80 percent of patients, 68 percent of physicians), to discuss personal fears (61 percent and 88 percent, respectively), to meet with a clergy member (69 percent and 60 percent, respectively), to have a chance to talk about the meaning of death (58 percent and 66 percent, respectively), and to discuss spiritual beliefs with one's physician (50 percent and 49 percent, respectively). Note that these are tasks for the patient, and that they resonate with the *Ars moriendi*.

11. Several studies of patient populations have found that at least two-thirds of patients welcome physicians' and other health care professionals' inquiring about spiritual concerns at the end of life. Charles Maclean and colleagues surveyed 456 patients sitting in outpatient primary care waiting rooms. They found that two out of three thought physicians should be aware of their patients' religious and spiritual beliefs. Although only one in three thought their doctor should ask them about religious and spiritual beliefs in a routine office visit, seven out of ten thought such inquiry would be appropriate if they were dying ("Patient Preference for Physician Discussion and Practice of Spirituality," *Journal of General Internal Medicine* 18, no. 1, 2003: 38–43).

12. At the University of Chicago, we followed 3,141 general medicine inpatients and found that those who reported after hospital discharge that one or more of their health care professionals had talked to them about spiritual concerns had significantly higher odds, on four different measures, of being very satisfied with their hospital care. Moreover, this remained true regardless of whether or not patients said they had desired such a discussion (Joshua A. Williams et al., "Attention to Inpatients' Religious and Spiritual Concerns: Predictors and Association with Patient Satisfaction," *Journal of General Internal Medicine* 26, no. 11, 2011: 1265–1271).

13. After studying hundreds of dying patients, Steinhauser and colleagues wrote: "It may be useful to recognize that for most patients and families who are confronting death and dying, psychosocial and spiritual issues are as important as physiologic concerns. Patients and families want relationships with health care providers that affirm this more encompassing view." ("Good Death," 825–832)

14. Jeffrey Bishop et al., "*Fides Ancilla Medicinae*: On the Ersatz Liturgy of Death in Biopsychosociospiritual Medicine," *Heythrop Journal* 49 (2008): 20–43. See also Bishop, *The Anticipatory Corpse*.

15. Timothy E. Quill et al., "Last-Resort Options for Palliative Sedation," *Annals of Internal Medicine* 151, no. 6 (2009): 421–424.

16. *Nicomachean Ethics*, book 1, section 1, tr. W. D. Ross (http://classics.mit.edu).

17. Leon R. Kass, "Regarding the End of Medicine and the Pursuit of Health," *Public Interest* 40 (1975): 11–42.

18. "Bucket lists" in the *Ars moriendi* literature are different from those in Hollywood, where examining one's conscience, confessing one's sins, and seeking reconciliation with God and neighbor don't figure prominently.

19. "WHO Definition of Palliative Care" (http://www.who.int/cancer/palliative/definition/en/); emphasis added.

20. "Statement on Clinical Practice Guidelines for Quality Palliative Care," American Academy of Hospice and Palliative Medicine (http://www.aahpm.org/Practice/default/quality.html); emphasis added.

21. Quill, "Last-Resort Options," 421. The same terms are used by others to justify euthanizing newborns with spina bifida. See Eduard Verhagen et al., "The Groningen Protocol—Euthanasia in Severely Ill Newborns," *New England Journal of Medicine* 352, no. 10 (2005): 959–962.

22. "Preamble to NHPCO Standards of Practice," National Hospice and Palliative Care Organization (http://www.nhpco.org/ethical-and-position-statements/preamble-and-philosophy); emphasis added.

II The Substance of an Art of Dying

5   Ritual and Practice

M. Therese Lysaught

Despite five decades of concern, challenge, and alarm, the medicalization of dying in the United States has not abated.[1] Instead, it has accelerated at an exponential rate. In an incisive 2010 *New Yorker* essay titled "Letting Go,"[2] the surgeon Atul Gawande tells the story of Sara Monopoli, a 34-year-old woman who, when 39 weeks pregnant with her first child, discovered that she had incurable metastatic lung cancer. She delivered the baby; then, over a period of seven months, she underwent four rounds of chemotherapy, none of which had much promise of working. (As Gawande notes, "there is no cure for lung cancer at this stage.") During those seven months, she suffered a pulmonary embolism; the cancer metastasized to her brain (for which she underwent more chemotherapy); and her original tumors continued to grow despite all treatments, spreading from her left lung to her right lung, her liver, the lining of her abdomen, and her spine. She, her family, and her medical team fought the cancer and each new assault. Eventually found to have pneumonia, she died in a hospital.

Gawande maintains that this modern tragedy—this almost ritually scripted performance of agonizing, prolonged, costly escalations of technological intervention at the end of life—is replayed millions of times. Though many people do meet death at home, or in long-term care, or suddenly, or under better circumstances, one-fifth of deaths in the United States—and the majority of deaths witnessed by hospital-based medical staff—currently occur in intensive care units.[3]

This book joins the nearly five-decade attempt to analyze the causes of this historically recent and seemingly intractable medicalization of dying and to provide a constructive way forward by positing an ethical framework for dying well in the twenty-first century. Ritual and custom have historically played prominent roles in the art of dying. From the Middle Ages on, these were particularly well described by the *Ars moriendi*, and in fact such practices served as an armamentarium of sorts to fortify individuals and communities in the face of illness and to help combat the threat of death up until the twentieth century. It seemed plausible, therefore, that an art of dying could be reinvigorated by renewed attention to the rituals and customs associated with dying.

However, the turn to ritual poses certain challenges. The place of ritual in secular culture today is ambiguous. The notion of ritual is often associated with particular religious traditions and so finds an uneasy fit within the secular, scientific context of present-day medicine and often leaves bioethicists shaking their heads. At other times, ritual is understood as a matter of a patient's personal preference—something non-rational, affective, and/ or cultural for which space must reluctantly be made within the biopsychosocial context of contemporary medicine in order to honor a patient's autonomy. Such accounts often deflect attention from the highly ritualized nature of present-day medicine (including the practices of bioethics, which is often far more powerful than any religious ritual in shaping people's experiences of illness and dying).

In this chapter I will wrestle with that ambiguity. Careful engagement with the problems associated with a contemporary understanding of "ritual" is beyond the scope of this study.[4] I will not propose a new ritual for the deathbed, nor will I step back and simply propose a framework for ritual at the deathbed. Rather, by returning to the *Ars moriendi* tradition, I will outline important concepts that bioethics and medicine will have to engage if they are truly interested in crafting a new art of dying for the twenty-first century.

I take as a significant point of reference the *Ars moriendi* tradition that emerged in the fifteenth century and informed Western citizens' notion of a good death through the nineteenth century. By attending to the protocols and customs involved therein, a series of components of dying well emerge: communal structures, practices, and virtues. These loci will help us make sense of factors contributing to the demise of this tradition in the nineteenth century—factors that remain operative today, including a new geography of dying driven largely but invisibly by the onset of market economics. I then bring the *Ars moriendi* tradition into conversation with a recent proposal for a new practice at the deathbed: Daniel Callahan's vision of a peaceful death, outlined in his book *The Troubled Dream of Life:*

In Search of a Peaceful Death.[5] Yet in Callahan's proposal the wisdom of the *Ars moriendi* tradition runs up against constraints imposed by the methodology of bioethics—constraints that limit the potential of his insights. Although Callahan's proposal falls far short of dying well, his vision of a peaceful, tamed, or (perhaps more accurately) well-managed death may be the best we can do.

Customs Marshaled

What might a contemporary art of dying glean from the historical practices of Western culture surrounding the end of life?[6] It is not uncommon for historical accounts of a topic to picture a "golden age" from which society has fallen. The history of dying in Western culture, however, is somewhat different, insofar as the golden age, by all reputable accounts, stretches "back to the dawn of history and is only now dying out before our eyes."[7] The golden age is, perhaps, only two or three generations distant, so some aspects of the *Ars moriendi* tradition may be able to inform present-day practices.

The classic account of the social shape of dying appears in Philippe Ariès's magisterial study *At the Hour of Our Death*. In this section, I begin with Ariès and then proceed to the tradition of the *Ars moriendi*, examining it through the lens of practice and custom. In doing so, I discover three important aspects of practices at the deathbed: they cannot be abstracted from a broader nexus of rituals, customs, and practices; they are grounded in a framework of virtue and character; and they emphasize the necessarily communal component of a good dying process.

The Classic Deathbed Protocol

Ariès opens his account in the Middle Ages, at the midpoint of a historical trajectory that stretches from the ancients through to the nineteenth century. He argues that over this two-millennium time frame—amid cultural differences, sociological changes, and technological developments stretching across Europe—dying was "governed by a familiar ritual."[8]

Ordinarily, the dying were the principal directors of their own dying process.[9] Equipped with advanced notice of their impending death, the dying would initiate simple customs or protocols that structured their final hours or days. Certain bodily postures were assumed, and a script was followed.

The dying person began with "a sad but very discreet recollection of beloved beings and things."[10] Forgiveness was asked from companions and family members, who were in turn pardoned, commended, and blessed. After setting communal relationships right, the dying person would turn to God—asking for forgiveness and commending himself to the Lord, being absolved by a priest, and receiving viaticum.[11]

As artistic renderings of such deathbed vigils make clear, dying was a social and communal event. The rooms of the dying became public places, which members of the community—even strangers—would visit freely. The practices of mutual forgiveness and blessing recognized that, in order for a death to be good, the spiritual well-being of the community had to be addressed. By emphasizing the connectedness between the dying person and the community, the historical practices acknowledged that death was as much a "wound" to the local community as to the dying person.[12]

The Art of Dying

In the fifteenth century, the simple deathbed protocol of the Middle Ages deepened into a more extensive set of practices known as the *Ars moriendi*, the art of dying. Arising largely in response to the ravages of the Black Death and its pandemic aftermath,[13] the original *Ars moriendi* literature was essentially a set of instructions for dying well—"a self-help manual for the person who was dying. In times of plague, one could not always count on a visit by the priest. It was to be read (and perhaps memorized) while one was still in good health, but it was to be kept and used in the days and hours of dying."[14]

Allen Verhey, in his book *The Christian Art of Dying: Learning from Jesus*, provides a succinct overview of the six sections of one of the earliest works in the *Ars moriendi* literature, the *Tractatus Artis Bene Moriendi*:

The first part is a commendation of death. The second part warns the dying person of the temptations confronted by the dying and gives advice about how to resist them.[15] The third part provides a short catechism with questions and answers concerning repentance and the assurance of God's pardon. The fourth part offers instructions on the imitation of the dying Christ and suggests prayers for use by the dying. The fifth part counsels persons, both the sick and those who care for them, to attend to these matters as matters of first importance. Finally, the sixth part provides a series of prayers to be prayed by those who minister to the dying person.[16]

Clearly the practices of the *Ars moriendi* tradition are deeply religious—in fact, deeply Christian. The simple medieval protocol at the deathbed—a largely secular protocol with a brief role for the priest—is presumed and recedes into the background of the text; the focus is on spiritual preparation for dying and death. To "die well" meant not simply to die calmly, surrounded by family members and friends, but primarily to die with one's spiritual house in order.

The Art of Living

To get one's spiritual house in order is no simple task. Thus, the focus of the *Ars moriendi* literature quickly shifted from the deathbed backward in time. Christopher Vogt, in his book *Patience, Compassion, Hope and the Christian Art of Dying Well*,[17] writes that a turning point occurred in the early sixteenth century with the publication of Erasmus's *Preparing for Death* (1533), largely considered one of the seminal works in the genre. The *Ars moriendi* tradition, Vogt writes, seeks to train practitioners on "how to live one's entire life so as to be ready for death." The genre becomes "about the art of living as much as it is about the art of dying."[18]

Thus, preparation for a good death began well before the warning that death was imminent. The primary task of each person was to cultivate the virtues necessary to die well—faith, hope, love, patience, humility, dispossession, and the ability to forgive. The principal way to grow in these virtues over one's life was through Christian practices—frequent or daily examination of conscience, sacramental reconciliation, as well as remembering death throughout life, practicing charity and mercy toward others, and spending time with the dying.[19] Through these practices, one habituated oneself in the virtues and skills required for a good death; through ritual and practice, they became part of a person's nature, making it easier to exercise them on one's deathbed.

Nor was this a solitary task. Verhey's account of the *Ars moriendi* makes clear that communities were considered essential for nurturing and sustaining practices of dying well and caring for the dying. We see this in a text titled *Crafte and Knowledge For To Dye Well*. In its fifth chapter—well before we get to the deathbed—it calls upon friends and caregivers to help the dying person die well and faithfully. Verhey writes:

It complained about deceptive assurances of recovery, about "false cheering and comforting and feigned behooving of bodily health." It insisted that friends and caregivers tell the sick honestly of their condition, that they encourage the dying to make peace with God and order their affairs, making a will and testament. It urged that friends and caregivers do what they can to help [the dying person] engage in those practices that could help one to die well and faithfully, and among those practices it counted confession and sacrament and above all, prayer. And it suggested that the whole community, "all the city," should come to the aid of the sick and dying.[20]

The art of dying, at least until the 1800s, took a village, if not a city.

Thus, the protocol at the deathbed was located within a broader set of practices, sustained by communities, that preceded and followed it.[21] This wasn't a new development with the *Ars moriendi*. Ariès notes, for example, that "before [medieval knights] left for the Crusades without hope of return, they received absolution, which was given in the form of a benediction. ... This same ceremony would be repeated, perhaps more than once, after their death."[22] In other words, customs at the deathbed presumed, drew on, and reprised rituals, practices, and customs that shaped people's lives; they were of a piece and situated within a broader nexus of intellectual, religious, and cultural traditions. Equally, they segued seamlessly into practices initiated at the moment of death.

Conventions Lost

No one would dispute that the complex religious and communal approach to death and dying that shaped Western culture until and throughout the nineteenth century has largely been forgotten. Callahan observes that we have lost "all those attendant rituals, habits, and practices that were able to give cultural meaning to death, to give it a familiar place in public and private life."[23] Ariès marks the turning point at the beginning of the eighteenth century and notes that since the end of World War II "we have witnessed a brutal revolution in ideas and feelings ... . Death, so omnipresent in the past that it was familiar, would be effaced, would disappear. It would become shameful and forbidden."[24]

Any attempt to reprise an art of dying, or even to develop an ethical framework for dying well in the twenty-first century, must examine more closely the factors contributing to this revolution. Here I provide snapshots of two of the factors: market economics and a new geography of dying.

A New Geography of Dying

The *Ars moriendi* and the history narrated by Ariès presumes a particular role for the dying person. But by the middle of the twentieth century that role was lost, and the loss significantly compromised any attempt at an art of dying. Verhey explains how this happened:

When dying was moved to the hospital ... there were some profound, if unintended, consequences for the dying role. Most notably, it was simply undercut, replaced by the "sick role." ... The dying were no longer treated as if they were dying; they were treated like anyone else who was recovering from major surgery or a serious disease. You do not go to the hospital, after all, to die. You go there to get better ... . So, suddenly, no one was "dying" anymore. They were just "sick." That spelled the end of the "the dying role" with its rituals and community. All that was left was "the sick role" and, of course, death itself.[25]

Two immediate factors contributed to this elision of the dying role—changes in the causes of mortality and in the geography of dying. First, the nature of the dying process is now, of course, quite different. With infectious diseases being mostly a thing of the past in the United States, dying has become a long and lingering process.[26] The leading causes of death today are chronic and degenerative disease—heart disease, stroke, dementia, cancer—"in which drugging and narcosis effectively hide the biological events that are occurring."[27] Dying, therefore, is no longer a discrete event but can be extended over months or years. Those who accompany this process are accompanying something different than before.

Advances in modern medicine are largely credited for these changes. Yet Ariès and others recognize that the loss of the art of dying and its rituals began well before medicine began to be effective. What additional factors, then, precipitated this brutal revolution? Verhey alludes to one factor briefly in the passage quoted above: By 1950, the place of dying had largely shifted from the home to the hospital. This shift, however, had begun much earlier, as Rob Moll notes in his book *The Art of Dying*: "In 1908, 14 percent of all deaths occurred in an institutional setting, either a hospital, nursing home or other facility. Just six years later the figure had jumped to 25 percent. By the end of the century it was nearly 80 percent."[28] How do we account for such a radical change in such an important social practice? One answer lies in the radical economic revolution that occurred a century earlier.

Visible Effects of the Invisible Hand

The reasons for this shift in the geography of dying are many. Yet as of 1914, the conquest of infectious diseases and the advent of a significant array of effective therapies had yet to occur. Surgeries were at last aided by antiseptics and anesthesia, and accuracy in diagnosis did accelerate beginning around 1870, but for the most part truly effective therapies remained future realities. Nonetheless, by 1914, the profession of medicine had succeeded in its efforts to consolidate its authority and increase its market power—efforts that began with the establishing of the American Medical Association in 1846.

Contributing to consolidation of medical authority was a reconceptualization of the hospital that began around 1900. As Paul Starr notes in *The Social Transformation of American Medicine*, the number of hospitals in the United States increased from 200 in 1873 to 4,000 by 1910, and to 6,000 by 1920.[29] Then, as now, hospitals were expensive propositions, and Starr details how physicians—formerly with little reason to ally with hospitals—were incentivized to refer patients to hospitals in this period, for mutual financial benefit.[30]

But why would patients go? For Starr, one piece of the answer lies in the radical changes in communal and familial infrastructure wrought by the socioeconomic changes of the Industrial Revolution:

Changes in both the family and hospital affected their relative capacity to manage treatment of the sick. The separation of work from residence made it more difficult to attend to the sick at home. With industrialization and high geographic mobility in America, the conjugal family also became more isolated from the threads of kinship, and so fewer relatives were close by in case of illness ... . Also, urban growth led to higher property values, forcing many families to abandon private houses for apartments in multi-family dwellings, which limited their ability to set aside rooms for sickness or childbirth. A 1913 analysis of the decline of home care of the sick noted, "Fewer families occupy a single dwelling, and the tiny flat or contracted apartment no longer is sufficient to accommodate sick members of the family. ... The sick are better cared for [in hospitals] with less waste of energy, and their presence in the home *does not interrupt the occupations and exhaust the means of the wage earners* ... . The day of the general home care of the sick can never return." Industrialization and urban life also brought an increase in the number of unattached individuals living alone in cities ... . In England and America, many of the first hospitals to care for private patients were built with lodgers and apartment-house dwellers especially in mind.[31]

Thus, the late 1700s—a period Ariès characterizes as a turning point in the practices of dying—also witnessed the emergence of the Industrial Revolution and a new form of capitalism in England. The relocation of labor from rural communities to urban factories inflicted radical, often brutal changes in the infrastructure of families and communities.[32] The internal logic of capitalism reconfigured workers as efficient machines whose work must not be interrupted, even to care for the sick.

Economic changes are not simply objective and material; rather, as the economist Karl Polanyi writes in *The Great Transformation*,[33] economies are necessarily shaped by and forward powerful philosophical claims about people and society. Economies, politics, religion, social relations—and, we could add, medicine—are, for Polanyi, intrinsically embedded in one another. In his introduction to Polanyi's book, the economist Joseph Stiglitz writes that "rapid [economic] transformation destroys old coping mechanisms, old safety nets, while it creates a new set of demands, *before new coping mechanisms are developed*."[34] Thus, one could argue that a semiproximate but often invisible cause of the brutal revolution in the shape of dying was the rapid and radical economic transformations that occurred at the end of the eighteenth century. Two hundred years later—a short time within the history of human culture—that we remain shackled to deformed dying processes is due largely to the continued yet invisible effects of an economy that increasingly subordinates all aspects of human life to the logic of the market.[35]

A Protocol Reclaimed?

If the foregoing is plausible, an ethical framework for a new art of dying in the twenty-first century will have to consider factors not ordinarily within bioethical methodology—questions of the infrastructure of care for the sick (geography and architecture and structures of communities); and the fundamental relationships between economics, medicine, and bioethics.[36]

In this section I will suggest one additional shift that occurred at the end of the eighteenth century, one that should be seriously addressed in any attempt to craft a new art of dying: the eclipse of virtue ethics as the dominant framework for ethics. I will use a proposal for improving end-of-life care offered by Daniel Callahan to explore this shift.

Toward a Peaceful Death

In his book *The Troubled Dream of Life: In Search for a Peaceful Death*, Callahan makes a proposal for "a peaceful death," an approach to dying that he believes combines the advantages of the historic "tame" death and the benefits of contemporary medicine. For Callahan, such a death would have four basic characteristics: it would be accepted by the dying person, it would minimize pain, it would maximize consciousness, and it would occur within community. In his words, a peaceful death is

a dying that is accepted without overpowering fear and a death that has lost its power to terrorize ... [by] a self that understands that control over fate will pass from its hands ... . It should also be a death marked by consciousness, by a self-awareness that one is dying, that the end has come—but, even more pointedly, a death marked by self-possession, by a sense that one is ending one's days awake, alert, and physically independent, not as a machine-sustained body or a body that has long ago lost its mind and self-awareness. Equally, it should again be death in public, by which I mean a time when friends and family draw near, when leave can be taken, when the props and devices of medicine can be put aside save for those meant to palliate and assuage.[37]

Callahan's peaceful death bears great resemblance to Ariès's description of a tame death, at least formally. Yet the substantive content of the interactions between the dying person and those who gather around her, or of the dying person's reason for a calm acceptance of death, is left undefined.

How does Callahan envision the dying person arriving at the point where death has lost its power to terrorize? Here, his proposal echoes the *Ars moriendi* tradition. Callahan rightly sees that at the heart of the question is character. Again and again throughout his analysis, Callahan locates a source of the solution to the problems posed by contemporary forms of dying in the "interior life," in inward attitudes. Following Victor Frankl and others, Callahan argues that the primary location of self-determination, self-definition, and real control over the self is the inner life:

The idea of a right to self-determination and self-definition is surely not meant to preclude the shaping of our inner life. ... But that capacity to shape an attitude inwardly is not taken as the interesting or important or meaningful part ... . We do not readily talk about how to shape our interior life in the face of death, because we think its meaning to be private, not easily shared or explored with others. ... [But] what enables people to endure, and to do so with dignity and grace, is not their ability to change their circumstances, but what they make of them; and what they make of them turns *on the kind of people they are*.[38]

Thus, Callahan's peaceful death turns on the character of the dying person. How one approaches dying will, for the most part, be consistent with or result from the character and virtues the patient has developed over the course of his or her life:

What we truly need is the capacity to master our dying, which is not the same as controlling it. Mastery requires that our interior self be in charge of itself, even when death is coming and control over the body has been, as it must be, lost ... . How should I want to live in order that I may die well? ... How should I begin to prepare myself for self-mastery, for pain and death? ... What kind of person do I want to be in my living and my dying? ... How we die will be an expression of how we have wanted to live, and the meaning we find in our dying is likely to be at one with the meaning we have found in our living.[39]

Thus, mastery of one's dying is the last step in the art of living.

The Art of Dying After Virtue

Yet unlike Erasmus and the *Ars moriendi* tradition, Callahan stops short of providing content for the lifelong process of preparing for death. He doesn't specify at length which character traits will be necessary for a peaceful death; nor does he propose how people are to achieve such a character, or what rituals or practices would be necessary or even helpful for engendering such traits.[40] In other words, Callahan's wisdom and insight point him toward an answer to the problem of contemporary dying: that we need a new *Ars moriendi*. But Callahan's ability to embrace fully his own answer is limited by a set of intellectual commitments that he himself had a part in creating: the formal, procedural logic embraced so passionately by bioethics. Bioethics eschews the ability to determine the truth of any particular end or good, and purports, via the principle of autonomy, to provide procedures by which individuals may pursue privately determined ends. Bioethics claims that all it can provide is formal processes within which individuals and communities can apply their own particular substantive visions.[41] Within this framework, only two options are available for a new *Ars moriendi*: either it would invent a generic and putatively neutral "art of dying in hospitals" available to all patients, or it would call for medicine simply to make a space for individual patients to draw on rituals from their own traditions or invent rituals of their own making.

Callahan proposes the first option but tacitly recognizes that this approach cannot but fail. He argues in *The Troubled Dream of Life* that we Americans, in order to reform our dying processes, will have to create a "common view of death"[42] and a "new understanding of the self."[43] He recognizes that, despite claims about American pluralism, there is a dominant and operative view of death and of the "ideal modern self." He describes how these ends and norms are part and parcel of the often violent and dehumanizing "rituals" currently practiced at the bedsides of dying patients, in emergency rooms, in intensive care units, and in nursing homes. Equally, he acknowledges that changing these rituals—changing the medicalization of death and the violence inflicted on the dying under the auspices of medical care—will require new (and particular) understandings of death and the self.

Moreover, Callahan acknowledges that operative rituals and concepts don't simply promote individually defined goods of patients, but primarily embed, embody, and promote the goods of the current social order within each particular patient, within each patient's local community, and within the health care institutions in which they are practiced. After outlining his proposal for a peaceful death, he tellingly writes "I call such a death a 'moral good' because it allows us to achieve important personal and social ends."[44] To link practices surrounding dying to broader social ends confirms the interconnectedness of any particular ritual with the intellectual, cultural, and religious traditions of the time and the place. Thus, in order for a proposal like Callahan's to advance, a new art of dying will have to look beyond bioethics to an ethical framework more adequate to the task. The philosopher Alasdair MacIntyre has outlined such a framework in a groundbreaking book titled *After Virtue*.[45] As Ariès and others make clear, the *Ars moriendi* was and remains embedded in a virtue framework. A thorough account of virtue ethics and MacIntyre's contribution to contemporary understandings of this framework is beyond the scope of this chapter, but for present purposes two points must be made.

The first point is MacIntyre's insight into the dynamic relationship between character/virtue, practices, and social ends. To reprise his now-classic definition of 'practice':

By a 'practice' I am going to mean any coherent and complex form of socially established cooperative human activity through which goods internal to that form of activity are realized in the course of trying to achieve those standards of excellence which are appropriate to, and partially definitive of, that form of activity, with the result that human powers to achieve excellence [e.g., virtues], and human conceptions of the ends and goods involved, are systematically extended.[46]

Callahan, in invoking personal and social goods as the criteria for assessing a death as morally good, intuits this connection between practices, ends, and, as the *Ars moriendi* tradition recognizes, virtue. To envision and seek to achieve certain standards of excellence with regard to dying has historically entailed a coherent and complex cooperative social practice that has achieved such excellence by realizing certain intrinsic goods. In doing so, the communities' ability to achieve those goods, and their understanding of a good death, was extended. The skills needed to achieve those goods—skills cultivated by the practices—were the virtues. That these goods are *internal* goods or ends is also important. Readers of a certain age may remember a dystopian 1973 film titled *Soylent Green*. Central to it is a practice that looks much like Callahan's peaceful death—an experience to which many citizens look forward as a relief from the gray, grim realities of their day-to-day lives. In a plot twist, it is revealed that this somewhat elaborate, much-anticipated and intentionally peaceful dying process (initiated when the dying are fully conscious and free of pain) aims at an external good: the practice turns bodies into raw materials for the production of Soylent Green, a food for an overcrowded planet.

A second observation made by MacIntyre takes us back to the eighteenth century. In his historical account of the development of contemporary ethics, MacIntyre argues that virtue ethics, as outlined above, was the dominant moral schema for most of Western history. According to MacIntyre and Ariès, the virtue tradition and the traditions of the *Ars moriendi* map the same chronological period. For MacIntyre, it is the end of the eighteenth century, when Enlightenment philosophers attempted to replace virtue ethics with the philosophical precursors of contemporary bioethics, and it was the failure of that project at the end of the nineteenth century that caused moral theory to fragment into the emotivism and philosophical chaos that mark present-day moral discourse. This is also the point where Ariès sees the *Ars moriendi*—a thick instantiation of the virtue tradition—beginning to unravel. Both shifts are concurrent with the rapid socio-cultural transformation initiated by the attempted shift to a self-regulated market economy and the advent of the Industrial Revolution.

In other words, an argument could be made that our current dying processes, which many rightly understand as deeply deformed, are inextricably of a piece with particular ethical and economic schemas of recent vintage. What we require are not new "rituals" for the dying process but new *practices*—practices that can vibrantly acknowledge the goods and ends sought, the virtues required, and the role of powerful but largely invisible cultural factors, such as economics, in limiting or enhancing our ability to die well.

Conclusion

From Jessica Mitford to Philippe Ariès to Daniel Callahan to Atul Gawande, bioethics has walked alongside health care, watching—and perhaps abetting—the ever-increasing medicalization of dying. In seeking to move toward an ethical framework for dying well in the twenty-first century, this book places the challenge for change squarely in the hands of bioethics. How might this essay contribute to that larger project? I conclude with five observations and a constructive proposal.

First, any framework for dying well will require bioethics to take serious stock of the limits of its own formal, procedural methodology. Those committed to the project of dying well concur: such a project is a virtue-based project. If bioethics is to contribute to this project, it will have to re-invent its own ethical framework to incorporate properly a virtue methodology.

Second, to do so will require that bioethics learn how to facilitate—in a real and constructive way—substantive clinical and cultural conversations about goods and ends.[47] Were bioethics to assist medicine in developing a protocol for dying well in the clinical context, serious questions would have to be asked about the social ends such a protocol sought to produce.

Third, bioethics will have to ask serious questions of economics, and not simply to tally the high costs of medical care at the end of life in a cost-benefit equation or puzzle over the challenges of who should pay for what. A serious ethical framework will have to attend to the myriad and powerful ways that present-day economic systems and philosophies quietly and often invisibly shape those who enter the clinical setting, determine the infrastructure within which patients and health care coexist and influence the biotechnology and health care industries.

Fourth, in addition to moving beyond the limited methodology of bioethics, an ethical framework for dying well will have to move beyond the clinical setting and reconstruct the geography of dying. If we are truly interested in reducing the medicalization of dying, the most logical step is to return dying to its proper, non-medical location: the home, or at least the local community. Looking beyond the ICU, how might health care practitioners and institutions help communities to care for the dying? Might congregations, for one example, reimagine how they care for the sick? Instead of sending communion ministers to health care institutions, might congregations repurpose vacant rectories as places to care for dying parishioners for whom home care is not a possibility?

Fifth, as the *Ars moriendi* literature ancient and new suggests, to focus on the deathbed is to miss the point. The art of dying is not simply a ritual that occurs after medicine has done all it can and "the props and devices of medicine [are] put aside."[48] From Ariès to Callahan and beyond, those seeking to reform the dying process make clear that practices at the deathbed must be related to a broader set of practices cultivated throughout life (and after death). The art of dying—which is really the art of living—is a lifelong process, cultivated in the home, in the congregation, and in the community. There the particular contents of different traditions may flourish, and the development of the virtues needed to die well (and, of course, to live well) may be pursued through specific rituals and practices accompanied by spiritual formation.

Allen Verhey proffers one of the most thorough proposals for such an art of living and dying in his book *The Christian Art of Dying*. As he makes clear, a contemporary *Ars moriendi* will entail a set of *practices*, understood in a MacIntyrean sense. These practices will be community specific and tradition specific, and will be practiced over a lifetime, by community members, for and with dying people, both for the dying and for the healthy—so that when the latter enter the dying process, they will be prepared to die well.[49] Any ritual at the deathbed will be one that caps this process, that flows from this broader set of practices.

Short of this, dying well or a good death will remain extraordinarily difficult to accomplish in the clinical context. At best, we may be able to move toward a tamed death—or at least a less medically malformed dying process. Following Ariès and Callahan, such a process would seek to do the following:

• make the dying the principal directors of their own dying process

• ensure that the dying know that they are dying

• enable the dying to take stock of their life, to express both gratitude for the goods of their life as well as sorrow for its closure

• integrate practices of reconciliation between patients, their family members and friends, and health care practitioners

• integrate patients' communities into the dying process

• acknowledge and tend to the wounds that death inflicts on patients' communities.

Would any of this—as minimal as it is—be possible within present-day medicine? Palliative medicine has laid the groundwork for such a tamed or well-managed death. But, building on Farr Curlin's assessment in chapter 4 of this volume, it may well be the case that dying is being deformed in new ways in the context of palliative care. A main question—and a question currently unavailable to bioethics—remains the question of ends. Were we to affirm this practice of a tame death, we would have to ask the question "Tame for whom?" Do we seek a tame death for the good of the patient, or for the good of the hospital and the medical staff? The "goods" sought don't have to be at odds, but they probably will differ. Insofar as the nature of those goods and ends will necessarily shape the practices and protocols themselves, it will be important to ask whether the protocols serve primarily the patients or the institutions.

Notes

1. See, for example, Jessica Mitford, *The American Way of Death* (Buccaneer Books, 1993; originally published by Crest Books in 1964); Philippe Ariès, *Western Attitudes Toward Death from the Middle Ages to the Present* (Johns Hopkins University Press, 1974); Ernest Becker, *The Denial of Death* (Simon and Schuster, 1973); Ivan Illich, *Medical Nemesis* (Pantheon, 1982).

2. Atul Gawande, "Letting Go: What Medicine Should Do When It Can't Save Your Life," *The New Yorker*, August 2, 2010.

3. Abraham Verghese, "Letting Go" (review of *Knocking on Heaven's Door*, by Katy Butler), *New York Times*, September 6, 2013.

4. For more background on the limitations of contemporary understandings of the notion of ritual, see Catherine Bell, *Ritual Theory, Ritual Practice* (Oxford University Press, 1992); Ronald L. Grimes, *Ritual Criticism* (University of South Carolina Press, 1990); Talal Asad, *Geneaologies of Religion: Discipline and Reasons of Power in Christianity and Islam* (Johns Hopkins University Press, 1993); and Arthur W. Frank, "For a Sociology of the Body: An Analytical Review," in *The Body: Social Process and Cultural Theory*, ed. Mike Featherstone, Mike Hepworth, and Bryan S. Turner (SAGE, 1991).

5. Daniel Callahan, *The Troubled Dream of Life: In Search of a Peaceful Death* (Simon and Schuster, 1993).

6. It must be noted that the *Ars moriendi* literature is culturally limited. Moreover, the topic of this book is extraordinarily specific to the US. The geography of dying and the causes of mortality in much of the developing world today remain the same as in the West up to the nineteenth century. It would be interesting to examine contemporary attitudes toward and practices surrounding dying in non-Western contexts, to see what we, in the US might be able to learn from our global counter-

parts. This process is known as "reverse innovation." See M. Therese Lysaught, "Reverse Innovation from the Least of Our Neighbors," *Health Progress* 94, no. 1 (2013): 45–52.

7. Philippe Ariès, *At the Hour of Our Death: The Classic History of Western Attitudes Toward Death Over the Last One Thousand Years* (Seuil, 1977; Vintage Books, 1981), page 5 of Vintage Books edition.

8. Ibid., 6. As discussed in the references in footnote 5 above, the analytic concept of "ritual" was established in the nineteenth century; thus, Ariès is using the term anachronistically here.

9. Not all deaths were ordinary or fit this pattern. Ariès helpfully discusses other situations—the death without warning (*mors repentina*) and the death of the saint. "When [death] did not give advanced warning," he writes (ibid., 10), "it ceased to be regarded as a necessity that, although frightening, was expected and accepted, like it or not. It destroyed the order of the world in which everyone believed; it became the absurd instrument of chance, which was sometimes disguised as the wrath of God. This is why the *mors repentina* was regarded as ignominious and shameful."

10. Ibid., 9.

11. Ibid., 14–18.

12. Ibid., 559, 603, 604.

13. Allen Verhey, *The Christian Art of Dying: Learning from Jesus* (Eerdmans, 2011), 80–86.

14. Ibid, 81.

15. Although there was some variations from tract to tract, the standard temptations in this literature were: to lose faith, to despair, to impatience, to pride, and to avarice or grasping after one's possessions (see ibid., 110–134).

16. Ibid., 87.

17. Christopher P. Vogt, *Patience, Compassion, Hope, and the Christian Art of Dying Well* (Rowman and Littlefield, 2004).

18. Ibid., 17.

19. Ibid., 22–29.

20. Verhey, *Christian Art*, 298.

21. Although Ariès's book is titled *At the Hour of One's Death*, the focus of most of the text is not in fact on the deathbed or dying process. The bulk of the 700-page book details practices that occurred *after* death, including funerals, cemeteries, and burial practices, tracing the shift from unmarked common graves and charnel houses to cremation and columbaria. Ariès's study reveals that even dead bodies are

sites of cultural production, reproducing in their decaying materiality the norms and commitments of their cultural contexts.

22. Ariès, *Hour of Our Death*, 140.

23. Callahan, *Troubled Dream*, 33.

24. Ariès, *Western Attitudes*, 85.

25. Verhey, *Christian Art*, 14.

26. This is, of course, not the case in much of the world, where infectious diseases, injuries, and accidents continue to be leading causes of morbidity and mortality.

27. Sherwin Nuland, quoted on p. 8 of Rob Moll, *The Art of Dying: Living Fully Into the Life to Come* (Intervarsity, 2010).

28. Moll, *The Art of Dying*, 15–16.

29. Paul Starr, *The Social Transformation of American Medicine: The Rise of a Sovereign Profession and the Making of a Vast Industry* (Basic Books, 1982), 73.

30. Ibid., 162–169.

31. Ibid., 73–74, emphasis added.

32. For compelling accounts of the powerful and violent effects of the economic destabilization wrought by the first waves of the Industrial Revolution on the poor and working class, and analyses of the philosophical commitments attending these changes and their social ramifications, see Karl Polanyi, *The Great Transformation: The Political and Economic Origins of Our Time* (Beacon, 1944) and Richard Henry Tawney, *The Agrarian Problem in the 16th Century* (Longmans, Green, 1912).

33. Polanyi, *The Great Transformation*, 1944.

34. Joseph Stiglitz, "Foreword," in second edition of Polanyi, *The Great Transformation* (Beacon, 2001).

35. "Deformed" is the term Callahan uses to refer to present-day clinical dying processes. See Callahan, *Troubled Dream*, 188.

36. I begin to address these connections in my article "And Power Corrupts ... : Theology and the Disciplinary Matrix of Bioethics" in *Handbook of Bioethics and Religion*, ed. David E. Guinn (Oxford University Press, 2006).

37. Callahan, *Troubled Dream*, 53–54.

38. Ibid., 129, 131, emphasis added.

39. Ibid., 147, 149.

40. Callahan does offer some character traits. On page 126 he writes "I want to invoke instead an image of the self that is more flexible, less manipulative, more

interdependent with others, more open to risk, a self appropriate to a peaceful death." He doesn't offer correlative suggestions of how these character traits might be developed, especially in a social context that shapes us toward the "ideal modern self" (120–121).

41. John Evans provides an excellent analysis of bioethics' adoption of instrumental, formal rationality in *Playing God: Human Genetic Engineering and the Rationalization of Public Bioethical Debate* (University of Chicago Press, 2002).

42. Callahan, *Troubled Dream*, 14–15.

43. Ibid., 126.

44. Ibid., 200.

45. Alasdair MacIntyre, *After Virtue: A Study in Moral Theory* (University of Notre Dame Press, 1981).

46. Ibid., 175.

47. Though this point doesn't follow directly from the foregoing analysis, any ethical framework for dying well must attend to the social location of this conversation. Much of the conversation on dying well rings very Caucasian, American, upper middle class, and male. Few data or narratives are drawn from communities of color or from lower socioeconomic tiers. Assumptions about the values that dominate end-of-life processes often sound quite gendered. And, as I mentioned earlier, the *present* dying process in *most* of the world is far from hyper-medicalized. We have an ethical and intellectual obligation to seek wisdom and insight from these "other" social locations, which are often right in the midst of our own.

48. Callahan, *Troubled Dream*, 54.

49. Rob Moll captures the power of this community-centered *Ars moriendi* for those who are not yet dying: "As anyone who has observed a good death can attest, it is in many ways a life-changing event for those watching. While tremendously sad and even horrible, a good death can also be beautiful and deeply moving. Such deaths were to be shared by members of the Christian community who were thereby encouraged in their faith. When death is public it is harder for the rest of us to become afraid of it. There is less mystery as we see how the physical body ceases to function. There is less fear as we see caregivers assist the dying in their last moments. There is more hope as we watch, even for a moment, the veil lifted and a dying person drawn into eternity. When we've seen a friend or loved one die, it's easier to learn to die. We can rehearse in our minds our own death, we learn what to do when others who we love face death, and we live better lives with eternity in mind." (*The Art of Dying*, 64) People so formed will probably behave very differently when they reach a clinical crossroads.

6   Spiritual Preparation

Michelle Harrington and Daniel P. Sulmasy

Reflect and see that the day of death is approaching.
Saint Francis of Assisi[1]

Contemporary American culture provides us with brief occasions to consider our own mortality, but these tend to be discrete and easily overlooked. A clerk at the Department of Motor Vehicles may ask whether one would like to be an organ donor. Funerals provide another obvious opportunity. In addition to the pamphlets scattered around the parlor advertising "pre-need planning," the memorial service may remind one of life's fragility and finitude. Unless the departed was especially dear, however, interment tends to mark the end of public mourning, and thoughts of one's own death are likely to be banished as one leaves the parking lot and returns to the land of the living. As Heidegger put it, in the everyday world "death is understood as an indeterminate something which first has to show up from somewhere, but right now is *not yet present* for oneself, and is thus no threat."[2] Thus, evasion, distraction, and denial rule the day.

Advance directives for health care provide another invitation for the consideration of one's mortality. But despite the alluring promise of extending the exercise of personal autonomy beyond the point of decision-making capacity—that is, of having one's health care choices honored after one can no longer speak for oneself—campaigns to promote living wills and advance directives have proved rather disappointing. Despite urgings from medical and legal associations, use of advance directives remains low; the elderly tend to delay their implementation and to show a marked preference for deferring to others.[3] While the creation of advance directives should ideally occasion important value-clarifying conversations about the end of life with one's loved ones, and, at minimum, designate a proxy for health care decisions, such legal instruments are necessary but not sufficient preparation for death. The literature of palliative care has recently moved from emphasizing these documents to a broader concept of "advance care planning."[4] Yet even advance care planning, as currently considered, is insufficient. As others have shown in preceding chapters, dying is not *only* a medical event, and although decisions about forgoing or requesting cardiopulmonary resuscitation or artificial nutrition and hydration are important ones, they are more fundamentally limned by the ultimate commitments of our lives and by our implicit philosophies and theologies of death.

The patient autonomy movement of the past several decades has aimed to secure a measure of personal freedom in the face of vulnerability, diminishment, and incapacity. With respect to the end of life, autonomy is posited as that which allows an individual to face death with integrity on his or her own terms. Preparing for death is thus understood as an exercise in antemortem preference satisfaction. In what follows, we seek to make explicit the connection between death and the freedom that the patient autonomy movement has correctly intuited as important. We will show, however, that the movement cannot secure the very freedom it has intuitively recognized as crucial and toward which it vainly strives. As theologians, philosophers, and sages have understood for many millennia, and as the *Ars moriendi* taught, dying well is a function of living well. In this chapter, we reflect on the concept of a spiritual preparation for death. In marked distinction to common secular accounts of preparation for death, we suggest that the life of a poor, sickly thirteenth-century itinerant preacher, who later became known as Saint Francis of Assisi, can illuminate the nature of death and the rather profound freedom with which it can be faced—if we don't dissemble and delay.

The Life and Death of Saint Francis

When Francesco Bernardone wrote to the mayors, consuls, magistrates, and governors of Assisi in 1220 enjoining them to "reflect and see that the day of death is approaching,"[5] he was following a medieval trope by reminding the powerful that death is the great leveler: high and low, rich and poor will be undone and dispossessed. His letter was undoubtedly a moral admonition and a goad to religious reform, but, true to his characteristic love and care for souls, it was also an invitation for the mighty to consider their pilgrimage on Earth with greater moral seriousness. According to their presumably common Christian faith, each of them would be called upon to account for himself on the day of judgment. By reminding them of their mortality, he invoked the great responsibility to use one's lifetime well.

Francis was just six years away from his own death when he wrote his Letter to the Rulers, yet he had begun to prepare for death years before. This preparation is depicted in many paintings, including those by Caravaggio and Giovanni Bellini, in which Francis, whether in a contemplative or an ecstatic pose, is depicted in the presence of a skull—a recurring artistic motif that serves as an ever-present reminder of death in the midst of life.

Francis was no stranger to asceticism. The skull represents many things, but its meaning includes the mortifications of the flesh to which he subjected himself, including frequent lengthy fasts and prolonged exposure to the cold. Yet in another sense, the skull represents the goal of his life: to die with and be conformed to Christ, to offer the substance of his life's history to his Lord, and to become, in a profound way, a true relic for his Order of Friars Minor and for all people of good will—an incarnate witness to the power and holiness of his life.

Francis remains among the most beloved of the saints. He is renowned for his voluntary poverty, simplicity, affability, care for the outcast, and blessing of the animals. The *legenda* (medieval inspirational stories) report that he was quite fond of the practice of removing his clothes to prove a point! While the hagiographic literature is both partial and vast, four moments in his biography can be seen to mark his pilgrimage through life and his increasing liberty of spirit: his early illness, his embrace of the leper, the receipt of his calling at the church of San Damiano, and his death.[6] Note that each point is an encounter with finitude, in himself or in another, and each marked for him a significant turning point. We will then analyze these aspects of his life in terms of theological and psychological understandings of death and generative life gleaned from Karl Rahner, Don Browning, and Erik Erikson. Finally, we will consider what all this might mean for "mere mortals" who don't expect to be canonized but nonetheless seek to face life and death with "alert hearts and open eyes."[7]

Early Illness

According to one biographer of Francis, Omer Englebert, those who knew him affirmed that he "never had any health."[8] He nevertheless had big dreams. As the son of a wealthy cloth merchant, young Francesco Bernardone had reasonable hope of upward social mobility, and dreamed of a valorous knighthood. He fought bravely to defend Assisi from Perugia's aggressions in the battle of San Giovanni, and was captured in 1202. He languished in a Perugian prison for nearly a year, where he bore his long captivity with humor and buoyant hopefulness, but fell gravely ill sometime after his release. Bedridden for several weeks, he required intensive care. This acute episode is only briefly relayed in the accounts of both Englebert and Bonaventure, but the brush with mortality seems to have been a turning point in Francis's life. He had been in mortal danger, and recovery had not been certain. When the threat had passed, he saw the world with new eyes. According to Bonaventure, affliction had enlightened his spiritual awareness.[9] Pleasant sights that once had made him happy lost their charm. For a while he was able to shake off this incident, and he quickly returned to his pursuit of glory, set on gathering the expensive accoutrement of knighthood. The costs of a coat of mail, lance, a flowing robe, an armored horse, and a squire were prohibitive for many a would-be knight. Yet in the midst of his eager preparations, he met a poor and badly clothed knight of noble lineage. Beset with compassion for his neediness and embarrassment, he promptly clothed the knight with his own fine garments that, up to that moment, held so much promise for his own longed-for future. In an instant, an empathic impulse had prompted him to relinquish what he had wanted for himself.

Hagiographers count Francis's early illness as preparation for his conversion to a life of resolute Christian poverty. Perhaps his appreciation for others' care of him during his time of need had stoked his own empathy for others, even as his illness had subtly effected a re-evaluation of his values and a reordering of his desires. Acute illness seems to have disrupted Francis's life plan, but his openness to and embrace of the disruption marked the beginning of the life for which he is famed. He began to live into the understanding of what it would mean to become a "knight of Christ" and to pursue a life of spiritual perfection expressed through the love of his neediest neighbors.

Embracing the Leper

Before embracing a life of poverty, Francis had been a dandy—a popular, carefree, well-dressed, cheerful young man. He had a horror of lepers.

With "putrefying flesh, oozing ulcers, and pestilential odor," they inspired instinctive fear and revulsion, and Francis had gone to extensive lengths to avoid them, sending others in his stead to take them alms.[10] His anxieties about deformity and diminution had even extended to a hunchbacked woman he had seen. As he experimented with a life of poverty, he began to fear that by continuing to mingle with beggars he would become like them[11]—an impulse that was, perhaps, more prophetic than paranoid.[12]

One day, as the *legenda* recount, Francis was riding his horse through the plain below Assisi when he suddenly encountered a man afflicted with leprosy. He experienced an urge to flee, but then remembered his vow to be perfect and recalled the self-discipline required if he was to conquer himself in order to be "a knight of Christ." Tenderly, he embraced the man, gave him an alms, and kissed him on his festering cheek. He felt a great happiness pervade his being, and in an instant his conversion was clinched: the object of his fear became the subject of his love and devotion.

Francis immediately began to seek out the lepers he had once worked so hard to avoid. He drew near to the afflicted in a neighboring lazaret, where he begged forgiveness for his former behavior and distributed more alms and kisses. According to Bonaventure, he went to live with the lepers outside Gubbio, where he served them diligently for God's sake, washing their feet, bandaging their ulcers, drawing the pus from their wounds, washing out the diseased matter, and lavishing kisses on their stigmatizing wounds.[13] This intimate, incarnational contact met the practical needs of the outcast afflicted and reintegrated them into the community of God. Francis, having experienced the perfect love that casts out fear, was emboldened to participate in the healing and building up of the world.

Receiving the Call

Francis's next act of building was quite literal—initially, at least. While kneeling in the dilapidated church of San Damiano, before a cross bearing a painting of the suffering Christ, he is said to have heard Christ say "Francis, go and repair my house which, as you see, is falling completely into ruin."[14] It is sometimes overlooked that the very image of Christ who gave him this command, was bleeding, broken in body, dying, and hanging from the roof of a ruined church. Francis hastened to obey the voice of this injured and suffering savior, and sold his worldly possessions to raise funds for the repairs. The church's priest, however, would not accept the proceeds for fear of drawing the ire of Francis's father. The priest was prescient; Francis's father *was* infuriated, and before long Francis appeared before the Bishop of Assisi and the townspeople to give back the proceeds and to renounce his father along with the goods that came from him. In characteristic fashion, he dramatically gave back his clothes, too, and stood nearly naked in front of the crowd. Having publicly affirmed his vow of poverty, Francis went on to beg for the money and materials with which to repair the church.

In typical hands-on fashion, Francis hauled stones and balanced on scaffolds to renovate San Damiano while he recruited help from whomever he could. Once the repairs were finished, he set out to restore the church of St. Peter, and after that the church of St. Mary of the Angels at Portiuncula. According to his biographers, he had, in the course of his exertions, come to understand the deeper meaning of the command to "repair Christ's house." He would go on to found three orders analogous to the three reconstructed churches—orders that would become known for voluntary poverty and self-spending love: the Friars Minor, the Poor Clares, and the Third Order. He would also develop a Rule based on the Gospel that would help to reform Christendom.

Francis lived for many more years, but ever in the shadow of the skull. His biographers convey a knowing dialectic of building and relinquishing, of adding friars to the Order, and becoming a spiritual father to many, but also of facing disappointment and losing control over the Rule by which he would have the brothers live. He pursued various forms of asceticism and made gains in self-mastery, even as he endured the consequences of his self-denial. He grew in conformity with the love of Christ and fervently desired to imitate Christ in his death. He thought he would win a martyr's crown by going to Morocco to preach the Gospel, but was thwarted in this aim just as he had been in his original pursuit of knighthood. He went in search of a violent death that would definitively allow him to display his steadfast courage and love of Christ, but instead received sickness and suffering, and had to be content with the grace of witness.

Sister Death

According to Bonaventure, God made Francis "remarkably renowned in his life and incomparably renowned in his death."[15] In the biographies, one sees in Francis a model of purposive activity until the very end—he aimed to "die in harness" as Christ's knight.[16] Francis sought to be of compassionate service to others, to care for his order, and to remain in intimate communion with God, even as he patiently endured terrible suffering. He died emaciated, blind, and in dreadful pain, after vomiting blood. Yet for all its gruesomeness, his death is remembered as beautiful. "In his dying, Francis showed other Christians how to die and how to care for the dying."[17]

On Mount La Verna, in 1224, Francis began to speak to his close companions about his impending death.[18] There he requested a season of solitude from the friars, and chose to dwell in a hut made of branches that he might review his life and repent of his sins, lament the divisions in his Order, and pray for its future. He held nothing back. In prayer he laid his life bare before God and freely exposed his grief, his doubts, and his sorrows. As he self-consciously prepared to meet his end, he struggled both physically and spiritually, but his sufferings were punctuated by periods of peace and joy and great intimacy with God—along with the companionship of a friendly falcon that visited him nightly. It was there on Mount La Verna that he prayed to know the pains of Christ's Passion and the love that impelled Christ to sacrifice himself.[19] From that point on, the biographies attest that he was marked with wounds in his hands, feet, and sides that remained for the rest of his life.

Francis bid farewell to Mount La Verna and took leave of the brothers there, knowing that he would never return. He traveled to Portiuncula on a donkey, in too much pain to walk. Even as he journeyed to meet his death, he healed others along the way. The *legenda* report that crowds thronged to touch the holy man, and to get their hands on anything he, or even his donkey, had touched. Along the way he stopped to rest at San Damiano, where he was cared for by Sister Clare and four of the brothers. There, where he initially received his vocation, he is thought to have composed part of the Canticle of Creatures, a profound expression of gratitude for and blessing of the created world. The song even took on a reconciling mission. When Francis learned that the civil and religious authorities of Assisi were quarreling, he composed another stanza and performed it in their presence to remind them of their common origins and dependencies, and of the blessedness of those who extend forgiveness to others. The little poor man, by then blind, was busy with the tasks of composing songs and reconciling people even as he prognosticated about his nearness to death.

Francis's "sickness unto death" lasted nearly two years; he saw several physicians during that time, including the Pope's. Their ministrations were mostly ineffectual, but he bravely endured a cauterization of his temples intended to heal his eye ailment. Another physician friend paid him a visit when his body became swollen with fluid, and Francis asked the physician for a prognosis regarding his dropsy:

"Brother," replied the physician guardedly, "I think that with God's grace all will be well."

"Please tell me the truth! For whether I live or die makes no difference to me. My great desire is to do God's will."

"In that case," replied the doctor, "I shall tell you that according to medical science, your disease is incurable; and my opinion is that you will die either at the end of September or the beginning of October."

Raising his arms to heaven the happy invalid exclaimed; "Welcome, Sister Death!"[20]

This exchange is remarkable on many levels. Like most good twenty-first-century physicians, Francis's doctor didn't want to destroy his patient's hope. He chose to use what might be regarded as an "indirect" style of communication. On a less charitable reading, he dissembled. Like many contemporary proponents of patient autonomy, however, Francis demanded the truth about his condition. He was prepared to hear it, to the point of embracing death as an intimate companion.

Friar Elias was reportedly scandalized by Francis's further preparations for death, which included expressions of exuberance and frequent singing of the third stanza of the Canticle of Creatures that he composed after his physician's prediction:

Be praised my Lord, for our Sister Bodily Death,
From whom no living man can escape.
Woe to those who die in mortal sin.
Blessed are they whom she shall find in Your most holy will,
For the second death shall not harm them.[21]

Despite his myriad infirmities, Francis claimed he felt so close to God that he couldn't keep from singing.

As his song indicates, Francis understood death as something inevitable that strikes from the outside. "No living man can escape" the death that finds each person in the patterns of his or her life. Though Francis clearly accepted and even welcomed this death, probably owing to the sense of preparedness that resulted from his season of self-examination and repentance, it is also true that he *enacted* his death. He offered his final testimony and blessings as provisions for the future order that would outlast his lifetime, and also practically instructed others to help him die a death that was fitting to his faith and in keeping with the life he had lived. Francis didn't deny death or its harbingers, and was therefore prepared to face his end transparently, in community with others.

When Francis's end was near, he asked to be taken to St. Mary's at the Portiuncula outside Assisi so that he could yield up his spirit in the city where he had received his vocation. As he was carried on his pallet, he instructed his companions to pause so that he could look out over the city and bless it. When he arrived in a wooded hut outside of the church, he asked to be placed on the ground naked so that he might, in the words of Bonaventure, "struggle naked with a naked enemy" and show that he was "going to Christ free and unburdened by anything."[22] Francis paired this dramatic bodily action with words of consummation and instruction: "My work is done. May Christ teach you to do yours!"[23] While his companions sang the third stanza of the Canticle, praising Sister Bodily Death, Francis offered forgiveness and blessings for those with whom he had journeyed throughout life. One friar lent him a cloak, and he was placed back on the pallet, where he then staged a para-liturgical feast, breaking and distributing bread to those present. His companions joined him as he intoned Psalm 41, and then he gave up his spirit. With hearts that were thankful for what they had witnessed, those present continued to sing throughout the night.

Theological Considerations

"Whenever someone dies freely," the twentieth-century Jesuit theologian Karl Rahner observed, "the whole of his life is present. This presence of the whole life, of the whole free spirit, commands our awe."[24] We are awed by the death of Francis. It is true that he died surrounded by those he loved, and by those who loved him. This is how most of us say that we want to die, and so his death, on that account, seems worth imitating. But that is hardly the whole story. Despite the suffering he endured in his last years and days, Francis's life didn't dribble out or trickle away; it was *consummated*—confirmed and sealed—in the death that he freely enacted. His dying wasn't simply "a part of life," as many present-day naturalists blithely recite. Rather, it instantiated what Rahner termed "the act of freedom."[25]

What, one may ask, has death to do with possibility or freedom, when it is colloquially lumped with taxes on account of its dreadfulness and inevitability? "[I]n the deed of the dying existence," Rahnerian theology replies, "man is necessarily free in his attitude towards death. Although he has to die, he is asked how he wishes to do it."[26] According to Rahner, each person has a fundamental choice to make about how to approach the mystery of death, which inevitably remains shrouded in darkness and linked with sin and human guilt.

One may adopt an attitude of autonomous defiance and deny death until the end, as did Susan Sontag. Upon learning that her bone marrow transplant had failed, she screamed at the medical staff, at members of her family, and presumably at the universe itself, "But this means I'm going to die!" She went on to seek and receive further experimental chemotherapy, which also failed. She spent her last weeks in a state that a psychiatrist called "protective isolation," almost unable to express herself. She kept taking the chemotherapy pills until she could no longer swallow them, then died in a hospital bed, wasted, delirious, septic, and in shock.[27]

Though Sontag's son has reported that this death was authentically hers—that, as a committed atheist with a strong belief in human progress, she fought relentlessly to maintain hope in her own survival—many, even atheists, will consider it less than ideal. She seemed to have achieved neither what Stephen Latham (in chapter 3 above) calls high values nor what he calls strong values. But Francis offers an alternative way to die—one that gestures toward the achievement of high values. His frank acknowledgment of his mortality, which allowed him to draw close to his companions even while taking his leave, demonstrates a path that can take one beyond the isolation of trying bravely but vainly to face death alone. Whereas Susan Sontag may have been known for embracing life with unflinching candor, Francis shows that it is possible to face both life and death with equal candor, acknowledging both the beauty and the finitude of life. Francis also points out how hope in human progress, however good, is never enough to satisfy the human spirit, which can be satisfied only by something that is both greater than the human and already present in the here and now. The result for Francis was a death in freedom—freedom from isolation, falsity, and despair. That kind of liberation is possible for anyone.

The autonomous defiance of death is but one temptation a Christian might face. One might also choose to face death as a simple biological process of personal extinction, or even to welcome death with the expectation that one's spirit will be released from its material shell. According to the Catholic Christian theology embraced by Francis of Assisi, however, each of these approaches misconstrues the meaning of life and death and the nature of the human before God.[28] That theological understanding is rooted in concepts that all people ought to be able to understand, regardless of their faith or other beliefs. A human is a union of nature and person; death is an event that strikes the human being "in his totality."[29] Though death is undeniably a physiological event, it is also distinctly historical, existential, moral, and spiritual. Insofar as the medicalization of death obscures death's personal aspect by exclusively attending to the natural (biological, physiological) aspects of dying, medicalization reifies an incomplete view of the human person and obscures death's personal significance.

According to Christian theology, the Christ event is both salvific and paradigmatic. In the sacraments of Baptism and the Eucharist, Christians profess to practice "dying with Christ" in the midst of their lives—to remember how Christ laid down his life for them, and to receive the grace with which to love God and neighbor ever more freely and lavishly. These sacraments remind Christians of the paradox at the heart of their faith: one gains one's life by losing it, by giving it away, laying it down, giving one's time and the substance of oneself to others in self-spending love. Christianity views this as true freedom—the free choice to love and thereby leave behind the bondage of mundane self-centeredness. We see this paradox embodied in the arc of Francis's life and death: Francis exhibited more freedom, self-possession, influence, and intimate communion as he increasingly unburdened himself and gave his life away.

Francis's early illness taught him to receive the care of others graciously and prompted him to identify with, and to have compassion for, those who suffer. Rahner notes that early Church fathers considered illness *prolixitas mortis*—the extension of death through life.[30] While Francis sensitively sought to relieve the suffering of others and to allow his companions to help alleviate his own, he didn't deny the connection between illness and death, and so allowed his early illness—a hint at the very finitude Bishop describes in chapter 2—to refine and change him: when he gave the needy knight his own cloak, he opened himself to a new and more authentic mode of living.

Deformity and diminution, like illness, are reminders of mortality. Francis's fear of lepers and of the hunchbacked woman undoubtedly sprung from the root fear of death; afflicted individuals threaten to contaminate those who sit at a comfortable remove from their own mortality. This is why Francis's conversion—as well as his spiritual preparation for death—truly began with his embrace of the leper. In that radical act, "fear died and conviction was born."[31] Francis overcame his fear of death and found himself freed to live rather fearlessly thereafter, to embrace voluntary poverty, and to risk sacrificial love.

Death and dying are present throughout life, in the harbingers of illness, in time that grows shorter, in options that are increasingly constrained. Fear of death is, according to Christian theology, to be expected, and stems from the innate recognition that it should not be. Death entered the world with sin and remains a standing reminder of human guilt. One is free to ignore or to deny the intimations of death, and to face death unawares; one may disregard the moral seriousness of death as the end of one's own unique and unrepeatable pilgrimage. To do so, however, would be to contradict one's own freedom and to fail to realize one's own humanity. According to Rahner, "death has to be understood as an act of consummation ... which is achieved through the acts of the whole life in such a manner that death is axiologically present all through human life. Man is enacting his death, as his own consummation, through the deeds of his life. Thus, death is present in his deeds, that is, in each and every one of his free acts, the acts by which he freely disposes of his whole person."[32]

One is given a finite time, of unknown duration and bounded by a real beginning and a genuine end, in which to accomplish one's life's work and in which to make an offering of oneself. The Christian tradition has variously conceived of this span as a "pilgrimage" and as "gift and task." Francis is remarkable for the way he disposed of his person with growing gratitude for his existence and an increasingly profound extension of love and care for others—and for the universe.

Rahner doesn't deny that death—both at the end of life and in everyday encounters—is dark and "unmastering." But since Christ lived and died with a freely loving liberty, men and women may follow in his footsteps and face death with freedom, love, and (paradoxically) self-possession. Death is no longer only a consequence of sin or a natural event common to all people, but now may be effected as a "dying with Christ"—as an act of faith and trust and generativity that we see modeled in the life and death of Francis.

Generativity

The word 'generativity' was coined by the psychologist and psychoanalyst Erik Erikson, but, as theologians have recognized, the concept gives voice to a spiritual truth: the love of an individual can extend through time, even after a person has died. In a real and recognizable way, "love generates the future."[33] Erikson wrote of generativity as the stage in adult human development that is concerned with establishing and guiding the next generation. Though generativity is usually associated with the raising of biological offspring, wherein love and care literally engender new, loving persons, Erikson recognized that many of the most generative people the world has known have applied the drive more broadly: "the true saints are those who transfer the state of householdership to the house of God, becoming father and mother, brother and sister, son and daughter, to all creation, rather than to their own issue."[34]

As "father" and "brother" to many living today, nearly 800 years after his death, Francis is certainly numbered among the truly generative saints. Francis's way of life, along with the Orders that he founded, continues to challenge and to inspire both the powerful and the lowly the world over; his life created new and liberating possibilities for those who would succeed him. Though Pope Francis (Jorge Mario Bergoglio) surely has "his own work to do," twenty-first-century Catholics and other people of good will have been energized by the appeal to his namesake, manifested through intentional simplicity, freely loving care for the marginalized, and rejection of the trappings of prestige. The hard-won fearlessness of the saint lives on, and the boundaries of his continuing influence are still undetermined.

In today's parlance, "spiritual preparation for death" is often expected to occur in close proximity to the end of life, perhaps with some assistance from hospice workers or a hospital chaplain. However, until the early nineteenth century, and even well into the Civil War, Christians were enjoined to learn "the art of dying" and to prepare for a "good death" while still in health.[35] Lydia Dugdale describes this in some detail in chapter 1. Some late-twentieth-century theologians have worked to reclaim the wisdom of the more traditional view by attending to human faith development through mutually illuminating psychological and theological insights that locate the end at the beginning—they consider the virtues and tasks of the end of life a starting point for their reflections, and then consider the developmental crises that an individual must successfully navigate throughout his or her life to realize these.[36]

For Erikson, "integrity" is the virtue of old age. One hopes that, in the final stage of life, integrity will preponderate over despair, "the feeling that the time is short, too short for the attempt to start another life and to try out alternate roads to integrity."[37] Integrity and self-possession resonate in Francis's last words: "My work is done. May Christ teach you to do yours!" Through an Eriksonian lens, this expression of completion and consummation rested on what Francis had generated in previous "stages" of epigenetic development, in which higher and later stages of development include, carry forward, and restate the earlier and lower.[38] Francis's "good death" depended on his having answered the call he received at the Church of San Damiano. There he had established his identity in a definitive way—a feat that relied on his still earlier life experiences, including the fearless initiative with which he embraced the leper. After San Damiano, he subsequently lived out his identity, building the Order, establishing and maintaining intimate relationships with his brothers and sisters, and extending God's love to every person and every other creature he encountered.

In Erikson's paradigm, the challenges of adult human development build on the earliest infantile accomplishment: establishing a sense of basic trust over basic mistrust. The tasks of achieving a sense of personal autonomy and initiative follow in early childhood. In Francis's free, creative, and communal death, we see the virtues of each stage of his life included and recapitulated at a higher level of integration. This Eriksonian insight echoes Rahner's theology: "In every moment of the free, personal achievement of existence, the past becomes an inner, essential principle of the present and its acts."[39] Spiritual preparation for death thus occurs in the midst of life, as one pours oneself out for others in freely loving actions.

Francis prepared himself to face the dispossession of death through everyday acts of *kenosis* or "self-emptying." By voluntarily relinquishing prestige and denying himself throughout his life, he had achieved the self-possession with which to provide for the future. He had self-consciously prepared to offer all he had become throughout his life to God and to his companions. Francis comprehended the movement of his whole life toward the moment of death, and yet one sees that his style was hardly morose or macabre, but rather joyful, purposive, and oriented to the space and time of his pilgrimage on Earth. He was always conscious of the idea that he had been given time to gain profit.[40] Insofar as he experienced the dispossession of death as a "downfall," he actively cast himself by faith "into the hands of the living God" in a free and final act of self-determination.[41]

Francis's final words and his example attest to the integrity he had achieved in his life, but also to the virtue of his great generativity. Through his acts of reconciliation and forgiveness and through the trust that he placed in his brothers and sisters, he made provision for the future, extending his love and care through time, even as he transparently prepared to "welcome Sister Death."

In his book *Generative Man*, Don Browning explores the insight of generativity in a practical theological vein: to a large extent, people exercise generativity by caring for what they have engendered and by investing in the people and institutions that will succeed them.[42] They thereby continue to exert influence on the world after their deaths. Rahner develops this insight through an innovative theological speculation. He notes that in classical theological formulations, death is described as the separation of body and soul, wherein the soul is thought to lose its relationship to the body and, hence, to the world.[43] In *On the Theology of Death*, Rahner postulates that in death the soul might actually *gain* a more profound relationship to the world:

[T]he soul, by surrendering her limited bodily structure in death, becomes open towards the "all" and, in some way, a co-determining factor of the universe precisely in its character as the ground for the personal life of other spiritual-corporeal beings … the individual person, once rendered all-cosmic through death and no longer restricted by the limits of our present life might come to have, through the actions performed in this world, a real ontological influence on the whole of the universe.[44]

It is perhaps easy to imagine how saints who are remembered, celebrated, and even supplicated might "ground the personal life" of living people and perhaps even continue to influence the operations of the universe, but what of "ordinary" people who are soon forgotten after a few generations have passed? Rahner suggests that such generative influence is available to all, even to those who die quiet and forgotten. One's spirit doesn't pass away; rather, it passes beyond, continuing to influence the world through what one became during life and thus posited in one's death. Only the "becoming" passes away; generativity persists. One's freedom to determine oneself is exercised in matter and time, such that death renders life meaningful. It is the limit against which people definitively express their faith, hope, and love.

Lessons for the Twenty-First Century

The life and death of St. Francis remind us that "advance care planning" ought to be far more comprehensive than simply strategizing about how to die with a minimum of discomfort. A "good death" seems to require more than the fulfillment of one's treatment preferences. There are opportunities for spiritual growth at the end of life that the prudent patient ought not overlook and the caring physician ought not subvert.[45]

As M. Therese Lysaught also suggests in chapter 5, preparing to die well requires great virtue—courage to grapple with finitude as the condition of one's freedom, integrity to face the reality of the threat posed by illness and impending death, generosity in being able to see one's dying as a lesson and a gift to others, and compassion, both on the part of those who suffer and on the part of those whose care for the suffering reminds them of their own mortality. These virtues are not learned in hours or days, but must be practiced and enacted throughout the moments of one's life, in communion with others.

The increasing transparency that Francis manifested over the course of his life can inspire and instruct. Mary Petrosky sees Francis's frequent nudity as a movement toward greater openness, frankness, authenticity, and innocence.[46] As Francis came to the full stature of integrity at the end of his life and asked to be placed naked on the ground, he dramatically displayed that he no longer clung to anything and yet was prepared to offer all that he had become. Although we in the twenty-first century need not imitate Francis quite so literally, it is salutary to consider that Francis's companions knew where he stood and what he valued. He had fully revealed himself and become transparent to others. At the end of life, others will be forced to make medical decisions for many of us. Their judgments will be greatly enhanced, and their burdens eased, to the extent that we have become transparent to them, through explicit conversations about end-of-life care and the appropriate documentation, certainly, but especially through the way that we have lived out our values—with maximal integrity and consistency.

Despite the best-laid plans, death continues to resist human management. It is still experienced as dispossessing and "unmastering." This is perhaps nowhere more evident than in cases of progressive dementia (see also Daniel Callahan's chapter in this volume) that extinguishes human personalities long before bodily death. How could one prepare for such an eventuality? In a sense, dementia simply throws the dialectic between building and relinquishing into sharper relief; one may not consciously preside over one's own decline, so one must do one's best to prepare by offering the fullness of one's faculties at every stage of life, by praying for a faithful heart, and by making provision for those who will care for, and will succeed, one. Francis's example is relevant here: by practicing gratitude for all that one has received, by seeking and extending forgiveness, and by facilitating reconciliation, one prepares to face the harbingers of death that occur throughout one's life. Despite the dreadful manifestations of dissolution and decline, one can be confident that death will not have the final word. In an essay aptly titled "The Comfort of Time," Rahner contends that, despite appearances,

one's past is conserved in the present of the person out of which arises every act by which a person really decides about himself as a whole in freedom.

Hence we can say: your whole life remains always preserved for you; everything you have done and suffered is gathered together in your being. You may have forgotten it, yet it is still there. It may appear to you as a pale dream even when you do remember what you once were, did and thought. All this you still are. All this has perhaps been transformed (as it is to be hoped) and incorporated into a better, more comprehensive framework, has been integrated more into a great love (indeed, the great love) and silent loyalty towards your God which was, remained and grew throughout everything life did with you ... .[47]

Death, as Francis demonstrated, is both suffered and enacted. Dark and dispossessing as well as revelatory of the human spirit, it introduces into the world what one has become in time. To "reflect and see that the day of death is approaching" is to prepare to live more fully and freely, and to give due consideration to the "order" that one will leave behind. One prepares to die well by practicing patience, humility, and self-spending love over the course of one's life. In the regular institution of the sacraments, Christians have the opportunity to attend to Christ's paradigmatic death and to prepare to craft their own. The sacraments may thus be appropriated as moments of grace and preparation in which Christian communities intentionally engage the mystery of death at the heart of their faith. Martyrs and those who, like Francis, have died "freely" continue to command our awe—they remind us that life's significance is not a function of longevity. The extension of one's love and care through time depends less on the number of days one receives than on one's willingness to use them well.

Notes

1. Francis of Assisi, "A Letter to the Rulers of the Peoples" (1220), in *Francis of Assisi: Early Documents*, volume 1, ed. Regis J. Armstrong, J. A. Wayne Hellman, and William J. Short (City Press, 1999), 58.

2. Martin Heidegger, *Being and Time*, tr. Joan Stambaugh (State University of New York Press, 2010), 243.

3. Angela Fagerlin and Carl E. Schneider, "Enough: The Failure of the Living Will," *Hastings Center Report* 34, no. 2 (2004): 32.

4. Linda L. Emanuel et al., "Advance Care Planning as a Process: Structuring the Discussions in Practice," *Journal of the American Geriatric Society* 43, no. 4 (1995): 440–446.

5. *Francis of Assisi*, ed. Armstrong et al., 58.

6. Daniel P. Sulmasy, *A Balm for Gilead: Meditations on Spirituality and the Healing Arts* (Georgetown University Press, 2006), 93.

7. Karl Rahner, *On the Theology of Death* (Herder and Herder, 1961), 17.

8. Omer Englebert, *St. Francis of Assisi: A Biography* (Servant Books, 1979), 23.

9. Bonaventure, *The Life of St. Francis*, tr. Ewert Cousins (Paulist Press, 1978), 187.

10. Englebert, *St. Francis of Assisi*, 32.

11. Ibid., 31.

12. Although Francis didn't himself become a "hunchback," he went on to experience severe disability and decay firsthand: he suffered from osteoporosis, the erosion of the bones in his extremities, and from chronic, ulcerated wounds in his face, hands, feet, and side. He was unable to walk in his final years and even went blind. For evidence that Francis contracted tuberculoid leprosy as a consequence of his close contact with lepers, see Joanne Schatzlein and Daniel P. Sulmasy, "The Diagnosis of St Francis: Evidence for Leprosy," *Franciscan Studies* 47 (1987): 181–217.

13. Bonaventure, *Life of St. Francis*, 195.

14. Ibid., 191.

15. Ibid., 321.

16. Englebert, *St. Francis of Assisi*, 249.

17. Sulmasy, *Balm for Gilead*, 98.

18. Englebert, *St. Francis of Assisi*, 238.

19. Ibid., 242.

20. Ibid., 268.

21. Ibid.

22. Bonaventure, *Life of St. Francis*, 317–318.

23. Englebert, *St. Francis of Assisi*, 270.

24. Karl Rahner, *Theology of Death*, 117.

25. Ibid., 93.

26. Ibid.

27. David Rieff, "Illness as More Than Metaphor," *New York Times*, December 4, 2005.

28. Rahner, *Theology of Death*, 52–54.

29. Ibid., 21.

30. Ibid., 83.

31. Joan Puls, *Every Bush Is Burning* (WCC Publications, 1985), as quoted in Rueben P. Job and Norman Shawchuck, *A Guide to Prayer for All God's People* (Upper Room Books, 1990), 322.

32. Rahner, *Theology of Death*, 51.

33. William Schweiker, "The Don S. Browning Memorial Service," *Criterion* 2 (2011), 13.

34. Erik H. Erikson, *Gandhi's Truth: On the Origins of Militant Non-violence* (Norton, 1969), 399, as quoted in Don S. Browning, *Generative Man: Psychoanalytic Perspectives* (Westminster, 1973), 145.

35. Shai J. Lavi, *The Modern Art of Dying: A History of Euthanasia in the United States* (Princeton University Press, 2005), 5. See also Drew Gilpin Faust, *This Republic of Suffering: Death and the American Civil War* (Vintage Books, 2008).

36. Browning, *Generative Man*, 181. See also James Fowler, *Stages of Faith: The Psychology of Human Development and the Quest for Meaning* (HarperCollins, 1995); Felicity B. Kelcourse, *Human Development and Faith: Life-Cycle Stages of Body, Mind, and Soul* (Chalice, 2004).

37. Erik H. Erikson, *Identity and the Life Cycle* (Norton, 1980), 104.

38. Browning, *Generative Man*, 22.

39. Karl Rahner, "The Comfort of Time," *Theological Investigations* (Helicon, 1961–1981), volume 3, 146.

40. Bonaventure, *Life of St. Francis*, 232.

41. Rahner, *Theology of Death*, 95.

42. Browning, *Generative Man*, 201.

43. Rahner, *Theology of Death*, 24–25.

44. Ibid., 31.

45. Ira Byock, *Dying Well: The Prospect for Growth at the End of Life* (Riverhead Books, 1997).

46. Mary Petrosky, "Praised Be My Lord Through Sister Death: A Franciscan Spirituality of Dying," in *Dying as a Franciscan*, ed. Michael F. Cusato and Daria Mitchell (Franciscan Institute Publications, 2011), 34.

47. Karl Rahner, "The Comfort of Time," *Theological Investigations* (Helicon, 1961–1981), 3: 147–148.

7 The Role of Community

Autumn Alcott Ridenour and Lisa Sowle Cahill

As more people supposedly choose for themselves the terms of their last days, often dying in institutions and separated from loved ones, communal identity finds itself increasingly absent from the bedside. However, an important question is whether people really choose where they will spend their last days and what health care they will receive. Are they capable of making such choices? Are they supported by loved ones and communities that aid and accompany them through the dying process? Grounding our claims in the Protestant and Catholic interpretations of the Christian tradition, we argue that any reinvigoration of an "art of dying" requires strong familial and communal relationships of care that "accompany" the dying in their final days.

Although this essay is written on the strength of Christian religious and theological approaches to dying, we trust that much of what we have to say will resonate with other religious traditions and with the experience of many medical professionals. Our essential message is that the human reality of death brings with it basic human needs, threats of suffering, and moral responsibilities that are shared across traditions and that require a communal response of "accompanying" the dying. Chaplains, pastors, and other religious advisors have a special role in meeting the spiritual needs of those rooted in religious traditions. However, the basic human need for accompaniment in the face of death should be a consideration in all ethical treatments of dying.

We argue that the definition of 'autonomy' need not exclude the role of community in end-of-life decision making. Instead, the notion of *relational autonomy*—that is, autonomy set in a context of community relations—corrects overly individualistic interpretations of autonomy that focus on self-determination alone. Drawing on insights from theological and philosophical understandings of autonomous agency that relates to one's social context evokes a sense of shared decision making and communal identity when facing end-of-life decisions. The implications for a revised understanding of autonomy are far-reaching, affecting how physicians, ethicists, families, and communities think about subjects such as physician-assisted suicide and the value of hospice care.

In order to understand the role that relationships play in constituting our individual identity or agency when facing moral decisions, we turn first to classic theological works in which Saint Augustine, Saint Thomas Aquinas, and Karl Barth establish a relational anthropology as constitutive of human personhood. Second, we consider alternative present-day autonomy arguments in the bioethical literature as they relate to physician-assisted suicide, particularly in the works of Tom Beauchamp and Ronald Dworkin. We describe how a retrieval of Immanuel Kant's original philosophical description of autonomy might amplify more recent interpretations of autonomy in the bioethical literature. Third, we explore contemporary Christian perspectives on human dignity, autonomy, and sociality in bioethics and end-of-life care. As these arguments, interpretations, and perspectives converge, we will illustrate in a few concrete ways how and why community support, including economic support, is essential to humane care of the dying.

Classic Christian Sources on Relationships as Constituting Human Personhood

Returning to Christian theological foundations allows us to see the full textures of a "relational anthropology" that grounds "qualified" autonomy in an ordered way. The classic Catholic theologians Augustine and Aquinas and the twentieth-century Protestant theologian Karl Barth ground human personhood in a context of embedded vertical and horizontal community relations.[1] Grounding human identity in relationships not only complements feminists' claims concerning "relationality" as pertinent to moral agency but also relates autonomy to the reality of "accompanying the dying" and a communal approach to physician-assisted suicide.

Augustine, Aquinas, and Barth all constitute persons in terms of participation in Christ. The beginning and the end of human existence reside in relation to God, the author and finisher of life. Living on "borrowed breath," we are created in the image of the relational Triune God, by which we are intended for ongoing relationship.[2] However, original sin reflects a broken interior relationship with the Creator that results in exterior or physical consequences, including the reality of broken horizontal relationships and physical death itself. In response to this problem, Augustine, Aquinas, and Barth, along with the whole of the Christian tradition, affirm the gift of the incarnation or God's becoming human in the person of Jesus Christ. Jesus Christ becomes the new way of relating to God that not only conquers the consequences of death through the hope of resurrected bodies but also provides a new way to be human by relating to Christ's incarnational presence as a divine and human person among us.

Through the incarnation, Christ reestablishes what it means to be human and a new way to participate in relationship to the divine life. Thus, we are created and redeemed for relation with God through union with Christ. This union extends to the *Totus Christus* or body of Christ as the covenant community existing in relation to God.

Augustine, Aquinas, and Barth write on death and suicide in a variety of ways. While Augustine argues that death was a result of the fall and original sin, he also affirms the goodness of the body as integral to human identity in a way that departs from the primary philosophical and theological interlocutors of his day, including the Neoplatonists, Manicheans, Stoics, and Christian Neoplatonists.[3] By affirming the good of the soul-body relationship, Augustine recognizes the great loss that occurs when death severs not only individual human identity but also human relationships and possible relationship with God. By affirming death as true loss, Augustine finds a way to legitimize human grief and the emotions associated with death that results in what might be called a new ethics of compassion.[4] Here Augustine acknowledges *timor mortis* or fear of death as natural and the comfort of Christ's compassion when Christ participates in human suffering.[5] This compassion is displayed through Augustine's interpretation of the Psalms, according to which Christ takes on the psychological anguish of forsakenness on behalf of the *Totus Christus* or body of Christ as a whole.[6] Christians are called to participate in Christ's compassion for the neighbor in need through service and friendship in ways that might accompany the dying through their experience at the bedside.

Likewise, Aquinas and Barth acknowledge the loss associated with death given the reality of human sin. Nonetheless, both offer hope through the resurrected life while also affirming the good in human finitude. Barth's theology, in particular, recognizes the dual tensions of loss and gift through the experience of aging and death.[7] For Barth, death involves both the negative consequence of sin and the good in human finitude. Thus, his ethics affirms the good in preserving human life but also accepts the reality of medicine's limits at the end of life.[8] Moreover, Barth's theology affirms the presence of a relational God in Christ, bolstering the role of a communal presence with the dying neighbor.

In addition, all three of these theologians address suicide. For Augustine, suicide reflects disordered love of self in relation to God and neighbor. To desire suicide is to neglect one's own existence as creature before God.[9] In this sense, to deny one's relationship to God and others is to overlook the mutual responsibilities and care existing within these relationships and, ultimately, to deny one's true identity. Likewise, Aquinas argues against suicide for three reasons: the good of self-preservation, the good of the part-whole relation whereby individuals are responsible to the common good, and the good of individual relationship to God.[10] Thus, relationships—with neighbors, with the community, and with the Divine—are integral to grounding individual self-knowledge and individual self-preservation. In this sense, the earliest understanding of Christian agency or identity includes a concept of autonomy rooted in relationships that reflect a covenant of care.

Barth nuances the Christian tradition in interesting ways. As James Gustafson notes, Barth helpfully acknowledges suicide as a forgivable act, though such forgiveness doesn't license the actions that preceded the act.[11] (In other words, the act of suicide might be forgiven after the fact.) Barth also recognizes "moral anguish" or emotional realities that distort rational perceptions for those contemplating suicide.[12]

On the other hand, although Aquinas and Kant recognize relationships as integral to the issue of suicide, their particular moral argumentation privileges the role of reason or rationality in this case, as in many others. Gustafson claims that Barth's emotional awareness is a welcome contribution to the discussion of suicide and of the end of life. In view of Barth's emotional sensitivity to moral anguish, his more personalist emphasis on one's relationship to God (behind the Divine Command) in preserving life is a welcome addition. Barth's contribution would be an important segue to contemporary medical ethics in its turn to the importance of care at the end of life while also acknowledging people don't look to medicine (or human institutions such as technology) in idolatrous forms.[13] Instead, a commitment to preserving life that also "allows death" in certain circumstances would remain the primary Christian approach to end-of-life care, thus maintaining a distinction between what present-day medical ethics describes as "killing" and "letting die." Thus, grounding decisions near the end of life in a context of embedded vertical and horizontal relationships would remain integral to theological approaches to medicine and bioethics, particularly as it relates to physician-assisted suicide and the principle of autonomy.

Present-Day Positions on Autonomy in Philosophical Medical Ethics

Interestingly, at least two extreme forms of autonomy appear to challenge current medical ethics. The first is the desire to preserve life at all costs by means of technology. The second (perhaps in reaction to the first) is to hasten death by approving physician-assisted suicide. Both aim to control death, either by prolonging life or hastening its end. Jeffrey Bishop argues that "decision" becomes the line between life and death or what is considered a "good life" or an "unworthy life."[14] Likewise, the bioethicist Daniel Callahan claims that the physical causality of death and its moral responsibility have been combined into one category within modern medical practice. Rather than attribute physical death to a biological reality, medicine operates under an aggressive mandate to intervene physically (even when the procedure seems to create unbearable harm), amplifying a cultural belief that humans are morally responsible for death rather than biology. From this perspective, traditional definitions of commission and omission become increasingly muddled.[15] The challenge posed to the traditional distinction between commission and omission is amplified by what Callahan characterizes as a fallacy on the part of social conservatives in their approach to modern medicine: they seem to believe "that a commitment to the sanctity of human life is best expressed and pursued through medical science and technological aggressiveness against death."[16]

Richard McCormick characterizes the desire for unending life through technological salvation as ironic: "Imagine a 300-bed Catholic hospital with all beds supporting PVS patients maintained for months, even years, with gastronomy tubes. ... An observer of the scenario would eventually be led to ask: Is it true that those who operate this facility actually believe in life after death?"[17] Similarly, in light of Ivan Illich's *Medical Nemesis*, Raymond Downing describes the idolatry of medicine in America as individuals' seek to preserve bodily life at all costs by means of technology.[18] On this analysis, autonomy is the desire to live as if biological life or vitalism were the point of living, rather than physical lives oriented to a spiritual end or relationship that ultimately results in eternal life with God. This form of autonomy appears to overlook the purpose of ordered love toward God that acknowledges the limitations of physical life: both in a faithful relationship before God and in healthy relationships with our neighbors.

Autonomy also becomes the ultimate good in philosophical arguments surrounding present-day moral and legal positions in favor of physician-assisted suicide. Tom Beauchamp strongly argues for eradicating the distinction between killing and letting die.[19] He argues that actions of omission and commission are morally the same, and that the actions of killing and letting die lead to similar results. For Beauchamp, because the physical end is the same, the means become morally irrelevant. Thus, he explicitly argues against the doctrine or principle of double effect, which is used to justify intending the good action while foreseeing two possible results, one good and one bad, without intending the bad result. In a traditional argument, the agent is considered to be directly responsible only for the good effect while the evil is said to be indirectly intended or tolerated.[20] For example, if a burdensome or futile medical treatment is refused or withdrawn, or if strong sedation is required to relieve pain, death may result sooner. However, alleviation of suffering is said to be the direct effect, and death merely accepted or secondarily "allowed," not directly caused. Euthanasia or physician-assisted suicide, in contrast, constitutes direct, intentional killing. They are morally excluded.[21] Furthermore, Beauchamp eliminates the distinction between ordinary and extraordinary treatment since treatment all depends upon the patient's wishes for its moral quality—whether prolonging life or hastening death—rather than fine discrepancies in direct and indirect intentions to bring death about. Instead, Beauchamp argues, the physical end, either hastening or allowing death, results in the same outcome: death. Thus, the means or actions leading to this end become morally irrelevant. What counts is the patient's choice. Offering an example, Beauchamp argues that all would agree that a physician performed a morally wrong action if he or she removed a ventilator from a patient who requested continued ventilation. Beauchamp concludes that the *real* moral decision lies with the patient and his or her autonomous choice to continue treatment, withdraw treatment, or hasten death by means of physician-assisted suicide. In this way, the patient exercises autonomy in the three possible scenarios. The physician merely accompanies the patient in the patient's moral desires or wishes as the patient exercises autonomy near the end of life. Likewise, Ronald Dworkin argues that moral decisions concerning end-of-life care ultimately hinge on individual autonomy.[22] In *Life's Dominion*, Dworkin identifies three primary components grounding the human person concerning questions at the beginning and end of life: beneficence, dignity (sacredness to human life), and autonomy (the ability to forge individual meaning within one's life narrative). However, Dworkin functionally subsumes beneficence and dignity under the heading of autonomy or the ability to pursue individual meaning in one's life. Moreover, Dworkin particularly fears dementia and the loss of one's rational faculties. He proposes two stages to autonomy in which the "rational" individual or "true self" anticipates and decides the outcome for the "irrational" or "secondary self" even when the secondary self may appear to find life enjoyable. Thus, Dworkin argues for permitting physician-assisted suicide in a legal context.

Although Dworkin's terms and mode of argument depart from Beauchamp's, their ultimate conclusions are similar in eradicating the moral differences between "killing" and "letting die." We disagree with their definitions of autonomy and with the possible upshot of their moral claims. For Dworkin, autonomy is primarily an issue of individual meaning-making and wishes made when one embodies one's "pinnacle" (able-bodied, rational) self. For Beauchamp, the moral onus resides with individual "autonomy" and with consequentialist reasoning. The same result occurs in direct killing and in letting die, so the end justifies the means.

However, Dworkin and Beauchamp depart from the notion of autonomy described in the philosophy of Kant in significant ways, Dworkin by prescribing a more libertarian notion of autonomy and Beauchamp by prescribing not only what appear to be libertarian justifications but also consequentialist reasoning. A return to a Kantian notion of autonomy will lead to a distinct moral framework and moral outcome.

For Kant, human beings are autonomous, self-legislating agents. The capacity to self-legislate is the capacity that distinguishes humans as moral beings. However, Kant's moral autonomy includes an important framework that balances individual self-legislation in a universal kingdom of ends. Kant's famous categorical imperative includes four principles: the universal principle, which includes acting in such a way that one's maxim is consistent as a universal maxim; the principle of humanity, which treats every individual as an end and not a means only; the autonomy principle, which acknowledges individuals as self-legislating individuals; and the kingdom of ends, where individuals forge moral maxims in accord with the universal kingdom of ends.[23] Kant argues against suicide on the basis of the second and the first of these principles. He argues that the principle of humanity includes the self; thus, in treating the self as an end and not merely a means, the individual has an obligation to self-preservation as opposed to self-destruction. Kant also argues that moral maxims should be universal. Suicide, like lying, couldn't be universally morally permitted, in that it would result in communal chaos. Thus, Kant argues against suicide. However, one could push Kant's own analysis further and argue that his universal kingdom of ends contains a *relational* component implicit within his own definition of moral obligations. The moral law is permissible insofar as the law proves to be universal in its possible application. In other words, Kant's understanding of autonomy includes an implicit communal dimension that recognizes a shared interest or law, the "universal kingdom of ends," that treats all people as ends. For Kant, autonomy is not a libertarian concept representing the sole individual's wishes, but a moral agency directed by universal laws that serve a community of shared ends. In view of this universal moral law, Kant's autonomy implicitly involves a relational component.

Edmund Pellegrino defends the standard distinction between killing and letting dying on the basis of intention.[24] Pellegrino disagrees with Beauchamp's insistence on collapsing the distinctions between ordinary and extraordinary means and between killing and letting die entailed by the principle of double effect. Pellegrino also considers a patient's choice in a more relational context and questions the implications of Beauchamp's position for the general practice of care for the dying. Pellegrino argues that Beauchamp distorts the physician-patient relationship by distorting the meanings of beneficence, autonomy, and trust within this relation. In terms of beneficence, Pellegrino asks who benefits: the patient, or the patient's neighbors? In terms of autonomy, Pellegrino questions whether or not the patient truly wants more choices. More choices lead to more anxiety, including the possibility that one perceives oneself as a burden in his or her particular community. Finally, Pellegrino argues that Beauchamp distorts compassion and mercy by allowing new choices that create anxiety for the patient left in a vulnerable relation to the physician. Such vulnerability might be greatly mishandled, and the new option of physician-assisted suicide probably compounds this vulnerability.

In other words, Beauchamp's and Dworkin's uses of autonomy involve a more libertarian approach whereby individuals are the sole source of moral decision making. This contradicts Kant's original notion of autonomy as set in a universal kingdom of ends in which the moral universal law binds all people in human community. In this sense, Kant's original autonomy involved an implicit relational sensibility that coheres in various ways with the role of relationships in Christian theology. Both Kant and Christian theology base moral decision making either on a universal moral law set in a kingdom of ends or on relationships with others, whether God or neighbor. Such relationships should prove integral to decisions made near the end of life in a context of community care.

Relational Autonomy, Community, and Care for the Dying in Recent Theology

When we approach care for the dying in our own time, we find the relational self, solidarity, and community reaffirmed in the recent Catholic and Protestant traditions of bioethics. Many medical professionals have arrived at a similar sensibility.

Catholic Resources

The sociality of the person and the person's constitutive relation to the common good are especially salient in modern Catholic social teaching, expressed in papal encyclicals from Leo XIII's *On the Condition of Labor* (1891) onward.[25] It is often said that the "twin pillars" of this tradition are the dignity of the person and the common good; far from mere autonomy, individual dignity is realized through social participation and by sharing in all the duties and benefits that constitute the good of society. The landmark document of the Second Vatican Council, the *Pastoral Constitution on the Church in the Modern World* (1965), affirms that "God did not create man for life in isolation, but for the formation of social unity" (no. 32). Thus "the obligations of justice and love are fulfilled only if each person, contributing to the common good, according to his [or her] own abilities and the needs of others, also promotes and assists the public and private in situations dedicated to bettering the conditions of human life" (no. 30).

Specifically addressing care for the dying, the Vatican's 1980 *Declaration on Euthanasia* considers, along with the value of the individual's life, the valid "desire not to impose excessive expense on the family or the community."[26] Yet the relation between patient and community goes two ways; family and community are essential to dignity, meaning, and happiness in one's last years or days. "What a sick person needs, besides medical care, is love, the human and supernatural warmth with which the sick person can and ought to be surrounded by all those close to him or her, parents and children, doctors and nurses."[27] As personal capacities diminish, others can help sustain a sense of loving embrace, reassurance, and prayerfulness. Families and caregivers necessarily assume much of the decision-making role in care of the dying. In Catholic tradition, bedside liturgies reinforce the relationship between the ill person, loved ones, and the church as a whole. In his 2012 World Day of the Sick message, Benedict XI emphasized "the sacraments of healing" (Eucharist, Reconciliation, and Anointing of the Sick), by which "the whole of the Church commends the sick to the suffering and glorified Lord so that he may alleviate their sufferings and save them." Conversely, by uniting themselves to Christ, sick people contribute to the collective good of the "People of God."[28]

Catholic moral theologians of the Post-Vatican II era follow suit. Correcting the ahistorical aspects of Karl Rahner's "theology of freedom" and his construal of the religious and moral life in terms of a "fundamental option," Charles Curran follows the critique of the political theologian Johann Baptist Metz: "The person as subject is a concrete, specific person formed in and through historical relationships and realities." Therefore, persons, their freedom, and their choices can never be "separated from concrete social and historical reality."[29] "The spiritual and moral life of the Christian involves growth in our relationships with God, the world, and one another," and "in working for justice and the transformation of the world."[30] In a widely cited article on seriously compromised newborns, Richard McCormick uses papal writings to back his belief that the true meaning of life lies in human relationships—relationships that ultimately lead us to God. Biological life exists, argues McCormick (citing Pope Pius XI), so that people may fulfill their "relational potential."[31]

The Catholic feminist ethicist Margaret Farley re-appropriates Kant.[32] She identifies shortcomings of the principle of autonomy in multiple settings, including the worldwide AIDS crisis and the care of the elderly. "When autonomy is narrowly construed in terms of total self-reliance, personal preference and self-assertion, it can compound the burdens of frailty and sickness that are experienced in varying and increasing degrees." Moreover, it can obscure "the more and more serious problems of distributive justice."[33] Farley's alternative is a principle and a disposition of "compassionate respect."[34] Compassionate respect involves a readiness to "suffer with" others, taking into account their concrete reality, including their specific needs and relationships.[35]

If humans are individuals who deserve dignity and who also flourish in relationships and communities, that implies that bioethics should attend to the moral dimension of the relationships between and among those larger spheres and individual patients. Supporting the idea of the natural sociality of the person with biblical sources, Charles Curran and Margaret Farley draw on themes and symbols such as "covenant" to establish the relational and communal dimensions of human beings and of biomedical care.

Catholic bioethics regards the responsibilities of religious, civic, and political communities to compromised or marginalized individuals, not least the sick. Communal care for the sick is a longstanding Christian ministry, evident in practices of hospitality in traditional religious orders and in Catholic and other religiously inspired health care systems today. The Catholic Health Association (CHA) of the United States, representing 2,000 Catholic health facilities, prioritizes "access to health care for all persons" and focuses "special attention on vulnerable populations who are unable to speak for themselves."[36] Karen Sue Smith writes:

In continuing the healing ministry of Jesus, Catholic health care tends to body and spirit, to the welfare of patients and their families, as well as to staff/employees .... . The church's social teaching—with its emphasis on human dignity, the common good, stewardship, solidarity, subsidiarity, care for the whole person, concern for the poor and vulnerable—also is made present, affirmed in the *Ethical and Religious Directives for Catholic Health Care Services*, in employee compensation and benefits, in charity care, and other ways.[37]

Today these "other ways" include advocacy for better, more inclusive health care services in the United States and advocacy for access to basic care globally as a human right. Reinforcing the CHA's advocacy stance, the *Ethical and*

Religious Directives published by the US bishops lays out the social responsibility of Catholic health care in terms of biblical care for the poor and the
common good of the entire society, urging that "particular attention should
be given to the health care needs of the poor, the uninsured, and the under-
insured."[38] In 2003, John Paul II targeted *"the very serious and unacceptable gap*
that separates the developing world from the developed" in terms of health
resources, and called for "justice and international solidarity" in order to
redress the balance.[39] The solidarity of community which the pope envisions
applies not only to the immediate family and caregivers of individual sick
people, and not only to their religious communities. He is calling for action
at the local, national, and international levels, involving religious organizations, civic groups, and advocacy networks and for international regulations,
policies, aid initiatives, and laws. As Pellegrino argues, the general ethos
in which care is provided is essential to a patient's dignity and well-being,
yet there is also a social justice component to care of the dying consisting
partly in the socioeconomic resources that are available. Compassionate care
requires a larger institutional infrastructure to support it.

Protestant Resources

Among Protestant theologians, churches, and international organizations,
a renewed trend to see bioethics in social and communal terms emerged in
the same era in which McCormick and others were making this same shift
from a Catholic perspective. In the 1960 and the 1970s, Paul Ramsey placed
strong emphasis on informed consent, but also noted that a great deal of
prudence or practical wisdom went into determining what adequate consent means concretely.[40] Therefore, the exercise of consent should always
be regarded in the context of bonds of that same loyalty and fidelity "that
is normative for all the covenants or moral bonds of life with life," speci-
fied in the peculiar relations of medical caregiving and receiving.[41] William
F. May similarly invokes the covenant between God and Israel to establish
the basis of Christian bioethics, and grounds the possibility of covenant
in universal experiences of human bonding within relationships.[42] Much
as Farley calls for compassionate respect for the particularity of patients'
situations, May argues that bioethics should be oriented toward the perspectives of those who receive care, rather than toward those of providers.
This necessitates a turn away from "dilemma ethics" (the primary realm of
the autonomy principle) and toward ongoing situations in which not all

problems can be solved and relationships of care and support are important.[43] James Gustafson, using the example of abortion, identifies "a Protestant ethical approach" as one that explicitly takes into consideration the
relationships, needs, responsibilities, options, and limits of those involved
in decision making, including primary agents, support systems, counselors,
and caregivers.[44]

Taking her lead from liberation theology, the feminist theological ethicist
Karen Lebacqz argues that the starting point of ethics should be the injus-
tices that inhere in relationships of exploitation.[45] As a North American,
Lebacqz attends particularly to forms of injustice that the privileged cause
or in which they are complicit. Comparing different approaches to bioethics, she highlights several values and insights from covenant ethics, virtue
ethics, care ethics, narrative ethics, feminist ethics, and womanist (African
American) ethics that are relevant both to human relationality and to care
of the dying. From a theological and a pastoral perspective, God's love must
be conveyed to every person, no matter what his or her state of disability or
decline. "But this love cannot be conveyed simply in the moment of crisis.
It is an ongoing task ... ."[46] The womanist Emilie Townes elucidates the very
specific conditions under which this "task" in relation to African Americans
is and is not fulfilled. African Americans suffer exclusion from the American health care system in myriad ways. For many African Americans, access
to hospice and palliative care is limited, and what care is available lacks
community-based integration with the continuum of care, both physical
and psychospiritual.[47] Yet Townes distinctively and strongly affirms that
both lament and hope are grounded in the agency of the oppressed themselves, in a divinely sustained collective energy that moves from despair to
accountability and the creation of new possibilities.[48]

Some major twentieth-century Protestant voices turned to a commu-
nity-ethic of virtue for the church and downplayed attempts to transform
society by enhancing the availability of more just and inclusive health
care practices, institutions, and policies. For example, Stanley Hauerwas
affirms a Christian vision of relationality as essential to human dignity, and
upholds the role of the community in supporting the vulnerable, including the sick and the "mentally disabled." Human dignity is not guaranteed
by any inherent characteristics, including the ability to make autonomous
decisions. The focus of Christian ethics should be on creating and sustaining the church in faithfulness to Christ's cross even in the midst of

suffering.[49] Yet Ramsey, May, Gustafson, Lebacqz, and Townes explicitly address policy and law. Attention to communities internationally and the global responsibilities of the churches rose to prominence in the second half of the twentieth century, in Protestantism as in Catholicism, increasingly prioritizing the "diseases of the poor," the major causes of death globally.[50] In the global South, care for the dying often means care for those enduring poverty, starvation, stigma, racism, sexism, and civil conflict. In 2009, the World Council of Churches helped to organize a Forum on Equity, Justice and Health, convening from around the world civil society organizations and social movements.[51]

Death and Practical Decisions about Care

Offering a detailed moral framework for care for the dying, Roman Catholic teaching proposes a difference between ordinary and extraordinary means, nuances the definitions of means to individual patients' circumstances, and calls for the availability of pain relief, palliative care, hospice, and above all, compassion, love, companionship, and psychosocial support to give life meaning even in its ending. Direct euthanasia is excluded, but morality doesn't consist mainly in prohibitions or in prolonging life as long as is possible. The focus is on "the right to die peacefully with human and Christian dignity,"[52] forgoing therapies that interfere with this goal, and accepting death as an inevitable part of the human condition. Beyond medical care for the dying, "how much more necessary it is to provide them with the comfort of boundless kindness and heartfelt charity."[53] In his apostolic letter on suffering, John Paul II calls for active support of others, especially near death, for "sensitivity, compassion, and help," exemplified by the Good Samaritan.[54] From a Protestant, biblical perspective, Allen Verhey concurs. Physician-assisted suicide cannot be "outlawed," but must be "out-loved" in the "more excellent way" of care at the end of life.[55] Death triumphs prematurely if and when patients are alienated from their own bodies, from their communities, and from God.[56]

Benedict XVI reiterated that the possibility and success of adequate support for the dying requires communal and social investment to create effective networks of care. He proposed to "support the incurably and terminally ill by calling for just social policies which can help to eliminate the causes of many diseases" and to support "improved care for the dying and those for whom no medical remedy is available," so that illness and death can be faced "in a dignified manner." For instance, it is "necessary to stress once again the need for more palliative care centres which provide integral care, offering the sick the human assistance and spiritual accompaniment they need. This is a right belonging to every human being, one which we must all be committed to defend."[57]

In a memoir detailing the trauma of the first two years after her 21-year-old daughter's sudden and devastating brain injury, the Catholic bioethicist Marilyn Martone provides a personal and compelling illustration of three ways in which care for the dying requires a relational and communal dimension. First, even when her daughter Michelle was unresponsive, apparently near death, or later cognitively and emotionally impaired, Martone was determined to be present to her. "The most valuable thing I seemed to be doing was sitting by my daughter's bedside and being present to her. There was no great exchange of ideas, no planning of a future, no decision-making; we just were ... . It was my presence and nothing I said or did that was important."[58] Perhaps a distinctive part of Christian care of the dying is assurance of personal presence for those abandoned by everyone else. This is central to the missions of Francis of Assisi (described by Michelle Harrington and Daniel Sulmasy in chapter 6 of this volume) and Mother Teresa of Calcutta, both of whom offered hospitality and care to the dying poor. When a dying person is confused, anxious, or semi-conscious, he or she can still be personally, spiritually and emotionally supported by those who remain near, attentive, and loving. In some sense, the community of care "fills in" for the declining capacities of the patient, sustaining his or her relationships, values, and spirituality.

Marilyn Martone states over and over that it was community that kept her going when she was exhausted, in constant fear of Michelle's likely death and the virtual certitude of non-recovery, and confounded by medical options and decisions. Friends and family members were important, but so was community forged with other patients' families and with medical professionals and hospital employees. "Even the hospital staff stops in to be with us because there is much laughter and little crying. They're practicing community, and I know that God is in our midst. We're our own little church."[59]

The support provided by a variety of specialists, medical facilities, nurses and nursing agencies, insurance coverage and Medicaid was essential to the level of recovery that was eventually possible for Michelle Martone. Marilyn Martone is acutely aware that her own education, status, and social knowledge brought protections and benefits to her daughter that weren't available to the children of other families also waiting, watching, and hoping in the same care facilities. An elevator operator who regularly brought Marilyn Martone fried chicken also had a daughter hospitalized with a head injury in the same intensive care unit. During a return visit after Michelle's release, Marilyn Martone inquired about her friend's child; the reply was "'She passed.'" She had choked to death in a sub-standard county rehab facility.[60]

Philosophical and Medical Perspectives

A good number of medical professionals and bioethicists, reflecting on experiences similar to those recounted above (their own or their patients'), are moving toward recommendations that converge with the religious and theological insights presented here. One medical resident reflected poignantly on a case in which she had been able to persuade the grandmother of a dying young woman that further resuscitation attempts would only add to the granddaughter's suffering. The patient died shortly thereafter, surrounded by family members.[61] Yet this same doctor was unable to convince members of her own family to cease last-ditch efforts to prolong the life of her 98-year-old grandmother in Taiwan.[62] Receiving an award from the American Society for Bioethics and Humanities, Eric Cassell turned away both from benevolent paternalism and from isolated autonomy, insisting that even freedom of choice implies background relationships. For ethics, relationships "are the basis of responsibility and the context of trust." Hence, the "ethics of individuals" must be supplemented by an "ethics of responsibility."[63] People never make decisions without the participation of others, and decisions by and about people with impaired decision-making capacity especially require the participation of families and of sensitive, well-informed caregivers.

A report on care near the end of life issued by the Hastings Center in 2013 arrived at guidelines nearly identical to those of Catholic teaching, including uses of the principle of double effect to justify refusal of life-sustaining treatment under certain circumstances and to justify palliative (terminal) sedation without directly intending death.[64] One difference is that the

Hastings Center Guidelines note the legal availability of physician-assisted suicide in some US states, neither approving nor condemning it, whereas the Vatican Declaration and the *Ethical and Religious Directives for Catholic Health Care Services* both rule it out absolutely. Where physician-assisted suicide is legal, communities have deemed it a support to humane end-of-life care. In the theological and relational perspective we have presented, physician-assisted suicide may be understandable, but ultimately it undermines truly compassionate and holistic care. A larger question, beyond the religious perspective, is whether compassionate care for the dying should prioritize support for the dying person in coming to terms with the end of life and in affirming or reconciling relationships with important others, over the termination of consciousness and direct termination of life. Appropriate pain relief would be part of supportive care, balanced with the need, desire, and ability of the patient to maintain some conscious relationships with loved ones and spiritual mentors. Farr Curlin addresses this is more detail in chapter 4 of the present volume.

Most important, the Hastings Center guidelines portray care for the dying and specific care decisions as collaborative processes that are highly reliant on institutional frameworks, established practices of care, caregivers' priorities and expectations, processes to facilitate decisions and mediate conflicts, legal protections, and socioeconomic policies that make resources available where they are most needed. Unfortunately, palliative care and hospice are not much more widely utilized in medical care today than when the first edition of the guidelines was published in 1987. Although hospice services are available in many medical facilities, and the percentage of terminally ill patients who die at home rather than in a hospital has risen in recent years, too many patients enter hospice care only a few days before death.[65]

Economics and Equitable Access

Although the Hastings Center's guidelines don't offer an ethical analysis of the American health care system or its reform, much less a justice analysis of the availability of care for the dying worldwide, they do acknowledge that the availability of resources affects decisions about care. "Developing an institutional practice of talking about the ethical dimensions of the cost of care aids in the development of policy to support the equitable allocation of limited resources. It also helps professionals with one of their most challenging problems: how to talk with patients and loved ones about treatment burdens that are economic."[66]

Knowing how to handle limitation of resources from within a health care institution is important. Changing the macro allocation system so that those who need care get it, or so that all have their basic needs met, is even more important, and extremely difficult. As Daniel Callahan describes in chapter 9 of this volume, families often are stretched to the breaking point in trying to provide adequate care and personal support to chronically ill, very elderly, or dying family members, and women bear the brunt of the burden.[67] It is important, therefore, for theological bioethicists and those engaged in religious health care ministries to engage with the "big picture" of care for the dying and to participate in work for change, as well as in theological-theoretical analysis. In so doing, theologians and other religiously motivated individuals and groups will partner with a variety of entities. This assumes that all those involved can agree on common aims and can cooperate on the basis of some shared understanding of what constitutes reasonable and equitable care at the end of life.

Anticipating the implementation of the Affordable Care Act of 2014, the Obama administration reached out to local government officials and civic groups to help publicize new insurance options and enroll new members, even in states with governors hostile to the reform effort. Of the 25 million Americans expected to gain coverage under the reform, 40 percent are Latino, which opens up a major opportunity for the churches, especially the Catholic ecclesial infrastructure and Catholic civic organizations, to help expand the reach of health care services. The chief executive of Dallas County in Texas made overtures "to the bishop of the Catholic Diocese of Dallas, to a lot of churches and religious institutions, and urged them to join our effort."[68] Having supported the Obama heath care reform program since its inception, the Catholic Health Association redoubled its efforts to expand coverage. At the national assembly of the Catholic Health Association, on its website, and in the CHA publication *Catholic Health World*, the CHA's president, Carol Keehan, urged members to advocate for Medicaid expansion in all states, and to enroll people in the new health insurance exchanges.[69] The CHA produced an informational video to facilitate the effort.[70] From a Protestant-inspired ecumenical standpoint, the social justice organization Sojourners advocates similarly for health care for all, including good care in dying.[71] In an article titled "Ethical Grounding for a Profession of Hospital Chaplaincy," Margaret Mohrmann discusses how hospital chaplains can be conduits of information and advocates within institutions for the availability of a variety of patient-centered services.[72]

Palliative care and hospice care may stand to benefit under the Affordable Care Act, and hence to become more available to those who are enrolled. Access may be expanded somewhat by the new provision that children may receive curative and palliative care concurrently, and demonstration projects for the same protocol involving adults are being proposed. In addition, one of the main purposes of the reform is to restrain costs by ensuring well-tested, appropriate, quality care, rather than quantity of services and procedures. "The field of hospice and palliative care is uniquely poised to be at the forefront of these inevitable changes, given the field's demonstrated ability to increase quality care at lower costs across all settings."[73] Palliative care and hospice improve health care's quality and reduce its cost while prioritizing the community support systems that enhance personal meaning and social connection for those in the dying process and their family caregivers. (See chapter 4 above.) According to Patrick McCruden, a vice-president of a Catholic health care system, Catholics motivated by the common good and preferential option for the poor, as well as others working in nonprofit health care, should take advantage of provisions of the Affordable Care Act to enlarge their ability to assess and serve community-level health needs.[74]

Conclusion

In this chapter we have presented a theological and pastoral ethic of care for the dying that emphasizes the relational nature of the person, the contextuality of autonomy, and the importance of a variety of community supports in providing responsible and just end-of-life care. We have also indicated how some philosophical understandings of the person and some contemporary nonreligious bioethical, medical, and policy approaches converge with our theological perspective. Finally, we note the importance of improving the availability of healthcare resources to enhance the dignity of the sick and dying. We urge theologians, bioethicists, and religious bodies to become advocates for, as well as analysts of, a just and compassionate community framework of care.

Notes

1. St. Augustine, *Confessions*, tr. Henry Chadwick (Oxford University Press, 1991); St. Augustine, *City of God*, tr. Henry Bettenson (Penguin, 1984); St. Thomas Aquinas, *Summa Theologica*, tr. Fathers of the Dominican Province (Ave Maria Press, 1981); Karl Barth, *Church Dogmatics*, volumes I–IV (T&T Clark, 1956–1975).

2. The term "borrowed breath" comes from David Kesley's two-volume work *Eccentric Existence* (Westminster John Knox Press, 2009).

3. John C. Cavadini, "Ambrose and Augustine: *De Bono Mortis*," in *The Limits of Ancient Christianity: Essays on Late Antique Thought and Culture in Honor of R. A. Markus*, ed. William E. Klingshirn and Mark Vessey (University of Michigan Press, 1999); Ambrose, "Death as a Good," in *Seven Exegetical Works*, tr. Michael P. McHugh (Catholic University of America Press, 1972). For further interpretation, see Autumn Alcott Ridenour, "Union with Christ for the Aging: A Consideration of Aging and Death in the Theology of St. Augustine and Karl Barth," dissertation, Boston College, defended September 2013.

4. Augustine, *City of God*, XIV, 551–564; Carol Straw, "Timor Mortis," in *Augustine through the Ages: An Encyclopedia*, ed. Allan Fitzgerald (Eerdmans, 1999), 839–841; Eric Rebillard, "Interaction between the Preacher and his Audience: The Case-Study of Augustine's Preaching on Death," *Studia Patristica* 31 (1997): 86–96, at 86.

5. Robert Dodaro, *Christ and the Just Society in the Thought of Augustine* (Cambridge University Press, 2004), 30–41.

6. Michael Cameron, "Enarrations in Psalms," in *Augustine through the Ages*, 290–296.

7. Barth, *Church Dogmatics*, III/2, 437–630. For further interpretation, see Ridenour, "Curse, Consolation, and Call."

8. Barth, *Church Dogmatics*, III/4, 427.

9. St. Augustine, *On Freedom of the Will*, III.vii–viii, tr. Anna S. Benjamin and L. H. Hackstaff (Prentice-Hall, 1964), 102–106.

10. St. Thomas Aquinas, *Summa Theologica*, II-II Q. 64.5, tr. Fathers of the Dominican Province (Ave Maria Press, 1981), 1462–1464.

11. James Gustafson, *Ethics from a Theocentric Perspective*, volume 2 (University of Chicago Press, 1984), 187–216.

12. Barth, *Church Dogmatics*, III/4, 403–410.

13. Ibid., 357.

14. Jeffrey P. Bishop, *The Anticipatory Corpse: Medicine, Power, and the Care of the Dying* (University of Notre Dame Press, 2011), 206–207.

15. Daniel Callahan, *The Troubled Dream of Life* (Georgetown University Press, 2000), 66.

16. Ibid., 72.

17. Richard McCormick, quoted in R. L. Fine, "From Quinlan to Schiavo: Medical, Ethical, and Legal Issues in Severe Brain Injury," *Baylor University Medical Center Proceedings* 18, no. 4 (2005): 303–310.

18. Ivan Illich, *Medical Nemesis: The Expropriation of Health* (Pantheon Books, 1976); Raymond Downing, *Death and Life in America: Biblical Healing and Biomedicine* (Herald, 2008).

19. Tom L. Beauchamp, "Introduction," in *Intending Death: The Ethics of Assisted Suicide and Euthanasia*, ed. Beauchamp (Prentice-Hall, 1996); Beauchamp, "Physician Assisted Suicide: A Response to Edmund Pellegrino," in *Choosing Life: A Dialogue on Evangelium Vitae*, ed. Kevin W. Wildes and Alan C. Mitchell (Georgetown University Press, 1997).

20. David Kelly, *Contemporary Catholic Health Care Ethics* (Georgetown University Press, 2004), 108–142.

21. Ibid.

22. Ronald Dworkin, *Life's Dominion* (Vintage Books, 1993), 24–29, 179–241.

23. Immanuel Kant, *Grounding for the Metaphysics of Morals*, third edition, tr. James W. Ellington (Hackett, 1993).

24. Edmund Pellegrino, "The Place of Intention in the Moral Assessment of Assisted Suicide and Active Euthanasia," in *Intending Death*, ed. Beauchamp.

25. See *Modern Catholic Social Teaching: Commentaries and Interpretation*, ed. Kenneth R. Himes (Georgetown University Press, 2005). All the papal encyclicals and other official documents are available at the Vatican website (www.vatican.va).

26. Congregation for the Doctrine of the Faith, *Declaration on Euthanasia*, 12.

27. Ibid., 9.

28. Benedict XVI, "Message of the Holy Father on the Occasion of the Twentieth World Day of The Sick" (http://www.vatican.va/holy_father/benedict_xvi/messages/sick/documents/hf_ben-xvi_mes_20111120_world-day-of-the-sick-2012_en.html).

29. Charles E Curran, *The Catholic Moral Tradition Today: A Synthesis* (Georgetown University Press, 1999), 97.

30. Ibid., 98.

31. Richard A. McCormick, "To save or let die: The dilemma of modern medicine," *Journal of the American Medical Association* 229, no. 2 (1974): 172–176.

32. Margaret A. Farley, "A Feminist Version of Respect for Persons," in *Feminist Theological Ethics*, ed. Lois E. Daly (Westminster John Knox Press, 1994).

33. Margaret A. Farley, *Compassionate Respect: A Feminist Approach to Medical Ethics and Other Questions* (Paulist Press, 2002), 29.

34. Ibid., 23.

35. Ibid., 39–40.

36. "About," Catholic Health Association of the United States (http://www.chausa.org/about/about).

37. Karen Sue Smith, *Caritas in Communion: A Summary* (Catholic Health Association of the United States, 2013).

38. United States Conference of Catholic Bishops, *Ethical and Religious Directives for Catholic Health Care Services*, fifth edition (USCCB, 2009), 7.

39. John Paul II, "Address to the Members of the Pontifical Academy For Life" (http://www.vatican.va/holy_father/john_paul_ii/speeches/2003/february/documents/hf_jp-ii_spe_20030224_pont-acad-life_en.html).

40. Paul Ramsey, *The Patient as Person* (Yale University Press, 1970), 3.

41. Ibid., 5.

42. William F. May, *Testing the Medical Covenant: Active Euthanasia and Health Care Reform* (Eerdmans, 1996), 94.

43. William F. May, *The Patient's Ordeal* (Indiana University Press, 1991), 3.

44. James M. Gustafson, "A Protestant Ethical Approach," in *The Morality of Abortion: Legal and Historical Perspectives*, ed. John T. Noonan Jr. (Harvard University Press, 1970).

45. Karen Lebacqz, *Justice in an Unjust World: Foundations for a Christian Approach to Justice* (Fortress, 1987).

46. Karen Lebacqz, "Bioethics: Eleven Approaches," *Dialog* 43, no. 2 (2004): 100–106.

47. Lavera M. Crawley, "Palliative Care in African American Communities," *Journal of Palliative Medicine* 5, no. 5 (2002): 775–779.

48. Emilie M. Townes, *Breaking the Fine Rain of Death: African American Health Issues and a Womanist Ethic of Care* (Continuum, 1998).

49. Stanley Hauerwas, *Suffering Presence: Theological Reflections on Medicine, the Mentally Handicapped, and the Church* (University of Notre Dame Press, 1986); Hauerwas, "Must a Patient Be a 'Person' to Be a Patient; Or My Uncle Charlie Is Not Much of

a Person But He Is Still My Uncle Charlie," *Connecticut Medicine* 39, no. 12 (1975): 815–817.

50. See, for example, Donald Messer, *Breaking the Conspiracy of Silence: Christian Churches and the Global AIDS Crisis* (Fortress, 2004).

51. "Documents Related to Health and Healing," World Council of Churches (http://www.oikoumene.org/en/resources/documents/wcc-programmes/justice -diakonia-and-responsibility-for-creation/health-and-healing).

52. Congregation for the Doctrine of the Faith, *Declaration on Euthanasia*, 11.

53. Ibid., 13.

54. John Paul II, *The Christian Meaning of Human Suffering* (http://www .vatican.va/holy_father/john_paul_ii/apost_letters/documents/hf_jp-ii_apl _11021984_salvifici-doloris_en.html).

55. Allen Verhey, *Reading the Bible in the Strange World of Medicine* (Eerdmans. 2003), 335.

56. Ibid., 337.

57. Benedict I, "Message for the Fifteenth World Day of the Sick" (http://www .vatican.va/holy_father/benedict_xvi/messages/sick/documents/hf_ben-xvi_mes _20061208_world-day-of-the-sick-2007_en.html).

58. Marilyn Martone, *Over the Waterfall* (CreateSpace Independent Publishing Platform, 2011), 132.

59. Ibid., 25.

60. Ibid., 200.

61. Guang-Shing Cheng, "Compromise," *Hastings Center Report* 37, no. 5 (2007): 8–9.

62. Guang-Shing Cheng, "Peace," *Hastings Center Report* 38, no. 6 (2008): 7–8.

63. Eric J. Cassell, "Unanswered Questions: Bioethics and Human Relationships," *Hastings Center Report* 37, no. 5 (2007): 20–23.

64. Nancy Berlinger et al., *The Hastings Center Guidelines for Decisions on Life-Sustaining Treatment and Care Near the End of Life* (Oxford University Press, 2013), 4–8, 183–184.

65. See, for example, Deborah Kotz, "Study Says Many Patients Enter Hospital Too Late," *Boston Globe*, September 5, 2013.

66. Ibid.

67. Meghan J. Clark, "Crisis in Care: Family, Society and the Need for Subsidiarity in Caregiving," *Journal of Catholic Social Thought* 7, no. 1 (2010): 63–81.

68. Robert Pear, "Local Officials Asked to Help on Health Law," *New York Times*, June 30, 2013.

69. Betsy Taylor, "Sr. Carol Urges Ministry to Stay Active in Promoting Insurance Expansion," *Catholic Health World* (http://www.chausa.org/publications/catholic-health -world/article/july-1-2013/sr.-carol-urges-ministry-to-stay-active-in-promoting- insurance-expansion).

70. "Ready, Get Set, Enroll!" Catholic Health Association (http://www.chausa.org/ affordable-care-act/overview#video).

71. See Julie Polter, "Living a Good Death," *Sojourners*, September-October 2010 (http://sojo.net/magazine/2000/09/living-good-death); Jim Wallis, "Faith Principles for Health-Care Reform," *Sojourners*, November 2009 (http://sojo.net/magazine/2009/ 11/faith-principles-health-care-reform).

72. Margaret E. Mohrmann, "Ethical Grounding for a Profession of Hospital Chaplaincy," *Hastings Center Report* 38, no. 6 (2008): 18–23.

73. Devon S. Fletcher and Joan T. Panke, "Opportunities and Challenges for Palliative Care Professionals in the Age of Health Reform," *Journal of Hospice and Palliative Nursing* 14, no. 7 (2012): 452–459.

74. Patrick McCruden, "The Affordable Care Act and Community Benefit: A Mandate Catholic Health Care Can (Partly) Embrace," *Kennedy Institute of Ethics Journal* 23, no. 3 (2013): 229–248.

III Special Considerations for an Art of Dying

8 Children

John Lantos

Parents whose children have been critically ill have written eloquent memoirs about their experiences. Alexander Hemon writes about caring for his daughter Isabel, who was diagnosed with a brain tumor.[1] He begins with a response that is common to many parents who are told that their child has a life-threatening disease—denial that it could be happening. He recounts how, when he was first given Isabel's diagnosis, his mind turned to irrelevancies rather than truly comprehending the enormity of the news he was receiving:

[The doctor] showed us the MRI images on his computer: right at the center of Isabel's brain, lodged between the cerebellum, the brain stem, and the hypothalamus, was a round *thing*. It was the size of a golf ball, Dr. Tomita suggested, but I'd never been interested in golf and couldn't envision what he meant. He would remove the tumor, and we would find out what kind it was only after the pathology report. "But it looks like a teratoid," he said. I didn't comprehend the word "teratoid," either—it was beyond my experience, belonging to the domain of the unimaginable and incomprehensible, the domain into which Dr. Tomita was now guiding us.

Lorrie Moore describes a similar experience when told that her baby had a Wilms' tumor.[2] She describes what it felt like when the ultrasound results came back (she writes in the third person, with herself as "The Mother"):

"What we have here is a Wilms' tumor," says the Surgeon. He says "tumor" as if it were the most normal thing in the world.

"Wilms'?" repeats the Mother. Among the three of them here, there is a long silence, as if it were suddenly the middle of the night. "Is that apostrophe s or s apostrophe?" the Mother says finally. She is a writer and a teacher. Spelling can be important—perhaps even at a time like this, though she has never before been at a time like this, so there are barbarisms she could easily commit and not know.

"S apostrophe," says the Surgeon. "I think. A malignant tumor on the left kidney."

Wait a minute. Hold on here. The Baby is only a baby, fed on organic applesauce and soy milk—a little prince!—and he was standing so close to her during the ultrasound. How could he have this terrible thing? It must have been her kidney. A fifties kidney. A DDT kidney. The Mother clears her throat. "Is it possible it was my kidney on the scan? I mean, I've never heard of a baby with a tumor, and, frankly, I was standing very close." She would make the blood hers, the tumor hers; it would all be some treacherous, farcical mistake.

"No, that's not possible, says the Surgeon.

The reason for these parents' denial is clear. As Hemon writes,

How can you possibly ease yourself into the death of your child? For one thing, it is supposed to happen well after your own dissolution into nothingness. Your children are supposed to outlive you by several decades, during the course of which they live their lives, happily devoid of the burden of your presence, and eventually complete the same mortal trajectory as their parents: oblivion, denial, fear, the end. They're supposed to handle their own mortality, and no help in that regard (other than forcing them to confront death by dying) can come from you—death ain't a science project. And, even if you could imagine your child's death, why would you?

The implications are less clear. How can they make good decisions for their children if they cannot even accept or acknowledge the diagnosis?

Hemon and Moore both explain, too, that it was almost unbearably painful to watch their children undergo invasive procedures in the intensive care unit. "In the ICU," Hemon writes, "we found her entangled in a web of IVs, tubes, and wires, paralyzed by Rocuronium (called 'the rock' by everyone there), which had been administered to prevent her from ripping out her breathing tubes. We spent the night watching her, kissing the fingers on her limp hand, reading or singing to her."

Moore, likewise, describes the powerlessness that she felt when she went to visit her baby in the intensive care unit: "It is a horror and a miracle to see him. He is lying in his crib in his room, tubed up, splayed like a boy on a cross, his arms stiffened into cardboard 'no-no's' so that he cannot yank out the tubes." Seeing him like that, she wants to rescue him from the medical torture that he is undergoing. "She wants to pick up the Baby and run—out of there, out of there. She wants to whip out a gun: No-no's, eh? This whole thing is what I call a no-no. Don't you touch him! she wants to shout at the surgeons and the needle nurses. Not anymore! No more! No more!"

Both talk about feeling utterly alone. Hemon titled his memoir "The Aquarium" because he felt, during the time when his daughter was sick, as if he was in an aquarium, looking out at all the people with "normal" lives.

"In the end," Moore writes, "you suffer alone. ... When your child has cancer, you are instantly whisked away to another planet."

Moore's baby survives. Hemon's baby dies. Their narratives capture the radical uncertainty and the tumultuous emotions that constitute parents' experience of a life-threatening illness in a child. As they were going through the experiences and making decisions, they had no idea whether the decisions were the right ones. Ultimately, the rightness or wrongness of those decisions would be determined by the outcome, an outcome that couldn't be known at the time that the decisions needed to be made. These narratives capture important components of the experience of death and dying in childhood today—uncertainty, helplessness, denial, fear of the future, anger at the doctors and the brutal nature of medical care today, and, ultimately, a profound sense of isolation.

Death was not always like this.

The Sentimental Death

Children often die in novels. In nineteenth-century novels there was a particular and unusual approach to childhood death. Deaths were sentimentalized in a way that made them seem to be pleasant and enlightening experiences. In *Uncle Tom's Cabin*, for examples, Eva died slowly and peacefully, taking care of those around her all the while. She was beautiful and virtuous, almost angelic. Everyone loved her and instinctively protected her. When Beth, in *Little Women*, died, a "beautiful serenity ... soon replaced the pathetic patience that had wrung their hearts so long."[3] When Dickens read the passage about the death of Tiny Tim in *The Christmas Carol* on one of his reading tours, the passage "brought out so many pocket handkerchiefs that it looked as if a snow-storm had somehow gotten into the hall without tickets."[4]

In these portrayals, childhood deaths were deliberate and anticipated. They were pain-free. There was never a possibility of, or questions about the appropriateness of, medical interventions. They are purified deaths written in such a way as to purify the reader with sentimental tears.

In the twentieth century, Dylan Thomas reacted against such literary portrayals. His enigmatic poem "A Refusal to Mourn the Death, by Fire, of a Child in London" confronts the excess of sentiment so prevalent in nineteenth-century novels. His refusal to mourn is a refusal to endorse or engage in the usual elegies of innocence and youth that accompany the death of a child. "I shall not murder the mankind of her going with a grave truth nor blaspheme down the stations of the breath with any further elegy of innocence and youth." His poem ends with a famous line about the singularity of death: "After the first death there is no other."[5] But even as Thomas reacted against the sentimentality of the nineteenth century, he, too, wrote of a death that was inevitable and unpreventable, not one that followed decisions about how aggressively to pursue life-sustaining treatment.

Changes in Childhood Dying

One striking fact distinguishes death in childhood today from death in childhood throughout human history: it is less common now. Before the twentieth century, at least 10 percent of children died. Almost all families and most parents experienced the death of a child; it was a near-universal experience.

As a result, mourning practices of the *Ars moriendi* variety were well known and commonly observed. Karen Rae Mehaffey studied mourning in nineteenth-century America. She noted that death was "a constant companion" to our forebears.[6] "Americans," she wrote, "were intimately acquainted with death. It impacted how people dressed, how they behaved in society, and even how they decorated their homes." There were, at that time, no funeral homes. Mourning ritual took place in the home. After a death, a black ribbon would be placed on the door to signal to the community that this was a house of mourning, while a white ribbon placed on the door would signify that the death was the death of a child. The mourners would wear certain clothes for prescribed periods of time. Everybody understood this set of symbols.

The fact that death in childhood used to be common led to different sorts of meanings for the death of a child than for the death of an adult. These meanings manifested themselves in the different mourning rituals that would be prescribed for childhood deaths. In some traditions, no mourning rituals were prescribed for the death of an infant. For older children, the period of mourning was shorter than that for adults. These reflected the social realities of mourning in a world where childhood death was more common and expected than it is today.

Many of these different responses carry over to today, even though the rationale for them—the commonness of childhood death—has disappeared.

For example, many people are uncertain whether to have a funeral for a baby who dies in the first days of life.[7] Many religions consider funerals or mourning rituals of any kind for infants to be unnecessary or at least non-obligatory.[8]

Today we have many more medical treatments to prevent illness in childhood than we had in the past. Thus, there are fewer fatal diseases and infant mortality is lower. Furthermore, for life-threatening diseases that continue to occur, there are many more treatments that can forestall death. Childhood death has become rarer, more unexpected, more unusual, and more difficult to predict. It has also become more deliberate. A century ago, and for all of human history before that, death just happened. Today, death almost always follows a decision to withhold or withdraw some intervention that could prolong life.

The transition from the historic norm of common childhood death to the modern era in which medical treatment could reduce mortality can be glimpsed in novels and short stories from the early twentieth century. In Sinclair Lewis's novel *Arrowsmith*, young Dr. Arrowsmith diagnoses a case of pertussis and races to the nearest druggist to get the antitoxin.[9] Diphtheria antitoxin was first used in the United States in 1894.[10] Arrowsmith was set in the early years of the twentieth century and published in 1925. In *A Country Doctor's Notebook*, Mikhaíl Bulgakov tells of saving a child with diphtheria by doing an emergency tracheostomy.[11] William Carlos Williams dealt with the same diagnosis in his short story "The Use of Force."[12] In each case, the doctors' practice had changed because of the availability of new medical innovations that transformed diphtheria from a commonly fatal disease into a potentially treatable one. The stories also convey the uncertainty that surrounded these new innovations. In *Arrowsmith*, the child dies despite receiving the antitoxin. In Bulgakov's story, it is surgery rather than medication that saves the child's life.

Together, these tales signal the change in pediatrics. With the advent of effective treatment came the need to decide when to discontinue treatment. We all must make choices that we never had to make before, in more circumstances than ever before. Often the choices must be made in circumstances of extensive prognostic uncertainty. People must decide whether to continue or forgo potentially life-prolonging interventions without knowing precisely how imminent death might be or even whether death is inevitable. Often they don't know whether or not interventions will be beneficial, harmful, or simply ineffective.

The ability to make decisions, to take action, to attempt to forestall death leads to a peculiar new phase in the course of a potential fatal illness. Today, patients, family members, and health care professionals must live for extended periods of time in what Barbara Sourkes has called "the living-dying interval."[13] "In the past," Sourkes notes, "the illness trajectory moved directly from diagnosis to death, with little intervening time or space. This 'new' middle phase can unfold in many guises: a cycle of remissions and relapses, a gradual downhill course, or prolonged remission implying a cure. ... The challenge which faces the patient and family is to maintain a semblance of normal life in the 'abnormal' presence of life-threatening illness." Stephen Latham makes a similar point in chapter 3 of the volume.

This "living-dying interval" characterized the period of patients' lives during which Dr. Elisabeth Kübler-Ross performed her groundbreaking studies on the ways that people think about their own deaths. Among her interviewees, "survival ranged from twelve hours to several months" "I emphasize this," she continues, "since we are talking about dying with patients who are not actually dying in the classical sense of the word."[14]

The living-dying interval can take place even before the birth of a child. A recent case in which obstetricians sought an ethics consultation illustrates this.

A Perinatal Death

The patient was a 37-year-old woman—call her Ms. W—who had been admitted to the hospital a day earlier at 28 weeks into a very complicated pregnancy. Ms. W had anti-phospholipid antibodies, a rare autoimmune disease that causes fetal heart disease and almost inevitably results in intrauterine fetal death in the first or second trimester of pregnancy. Ms. W had been trying desperately for decades to have a baby. This was her eighteenth pregnancy. The previous seventeen had ended in miscarriage.

This was the farthest along she had ever gotten in a pregnancy. But the fetus wasn't doing well. The fetal ultrasound showed that the baby had developed severe heart problems or "cardiomyopathy." Fetal death seemed imminent. Furthermore, the disease had led to intrauterine growth retardation. The obstetricians estimated that based on the ultrasound the fetus weighed only 290 grams. That is the average weight for a fetus at 19 weeks of gestation.

The doctors thought that the fetus would soon die and that there was nothing they could do to save it. They told this to Ms. W. She asked about the possibility of doing a caesarian section. The doctors felt that an operation would be too risky for the mother and would be of no benefit to the fetus at that extremely low birth weight. Ms. W wanted the c-section anyway because she wanted her baby to be delivered alive. She wanted to hold her live baby. The doctor asked several ethicists (the present author among them) whether we thought he should do the c-section, whether he had to do the c-section, or whether he had the right to refuse.

Often, ethics consultants must try to figure out what the real ethical question is before they can begin to formulate a solution or a recommendation. In this case, there seemed to be at least two things going on. One was the pure kick-in-the-gut pain one felt in listening to this woman's story, her odyssey, her desperation to have a baby. Eighteen pregnancies! One could imagine that, in the earliest ones, nobody knew what was going on and she was reassured that the next one would be okay. Then, as the number of miscarriages grew, and the doctors worked out the cause, there must have been years of despair and counseling that she should never try again, that she was incapable of carrying a pregnancy to term, that it was too dangerous even to try. And then, perhaps, she was offered a glimmer of hope with advances in perinatal care, a hint of a possibility that she might, someday, realize her dream of having a baby of her own. This set of concerns, however, didn't lead to a current ethical dilemma, though it probably did lead to a sense that this wasn't a typical case, a normal case, a case in which one could necessarily rely on one's moral intuitions.

Instead, the problem was with those moral intuitions. The doctors seemed troubled by the request for a c-section. There was a risk that, if they did the operation, they would harm Ms. W. She could even die. And the chances were infinitesimal at best that the operation would lead to the survival of the baby. So, in an "ordinary" case, they would probably have not been willing to do the c-section. But then there was that extraordinary history. This clearly was no ordinary case.

Good ethics start with good facts, so we looked for data.

C-sections, or any operations, clearly are more dangerous when patients have antiphospholipid antibodies. The medical literature showed that there was an increased risk of bleeding during the operation and perhaps an increased risk of life-threatening infection, or sepsis, post-operatively.

Nobody could say for sure how high that risk was, only that it was higher than in a healthy patient. The doctor's concerns about bleeding were somewhat based on a careful review of the published medical literature. But there was not much published in the medical literature. There were only a few case reports of complications after surgery. These suggested that the risks might be higher than for a patient without this disease but didn't allow a precise estimate of just how much higher they might be.

The data on survival for the baby was also just a bit ambiguous. Survival for a baby at 290 grams was virtually unprecedented. There had, however, been a few case reports. And they had always been in babies with intrauterine growth retardation, that is, in babies who were small for their gestational age and so, more gestationally mature than their birth weight would suggest. And there was always the possibility of some inaccuracy of the weight estimate by ultrasound, so we didn't know for sure how much this baby actually weighed. The only way to be sure of the baby's birth weight would be to take the baby out and weigh it.

Nobody would recommend a c-section under these circumstances. The question was whether we should forbid it.

We went to talk to the patient.

She was sitting in her bed with the fetal monitor ticking away at her bedside. The fetal heartbeat was regular. Her hands were folded across her belly. We introduced ourselves as members of the ethics consultation service. She had been expecting us.

Ethics consultant: We wanted to hear from you what you've been told about the risks of having a c-section and about the chances that your baby could survive.

Ms. W: They told me that, with the c-section, there is a 1/1000 chance that I could die. They also said that, without a c-section, she will certainly die.

Ethics consultant: Did they tell you that there was almost no chance that your baby could survive?

Ms. W: Yes. But it doesn't matter. It's her only chance.

Ethics consultant: Have you discussed this with your husband?

Ms. W: We've talked about it. He agrees. It's our last chance.

Ethics consultant: Your doctor is a little concerned that you will be at higher risk for bleeding during the operation than most women.

Ms. W: I told him that if anything goes wrong, he should save me first.

While Ms. W spoke, a few tears rolled down her cheek. We found some tissues for her. She wiped away the tears and shook her head.

Ms. W: I don't really feel like I have any choice. It's out of my hands.

Ethics consultant: Well, you do have a choice. You don't have to have a c-section.

Ms. W: What would you do?

As she asked, looking right at me, her eyes still moist but clear and direct.

Ethics consultant: I don't know, I said. I really don't know.

I noticed that during the conversation, Ms. W shifted in the way she described the basis for her choice. She began with a straightforward recitation of the facts—as if to prove to me, and perhaps to herself, that she clearly understood the prognosis. She even seemed to understand that the doctors considered those facts to be determinative of the right choice. But, for her, those facts meant something different, something less important, because she went on to put them in context. First, she said "It (that is, the data) doesn't matter." Then she said "It's her only chance." Then she said "It's our last chance." Finally, she said "I don't really feel like I have any choice. It is out of my hands." These words may have been meant symbolically. They may have been hyperbole. She may not have meant them literally. That is the way we usually hear and interpret such statements. We say "Well, she really *understands* that she does have a choice, she's just feeling as if she doesn't." Or we say "Well, she has weighed the physical risks against the emotional benefits and come up with a decision that reflects her own values." But it may be that she really feels like she has no choice, and if so, her own assessment of her own freedoms and obligations may give us some insights into the ways that parents think about decisions that might lead to the death—or the survival—of a critically ill baby.

Learning from Stories

These stories show us the ways in which the death of a child is different from the death of an adult. It is different because we tend to identify with the parents. But dying is a community affair—as the preceding chapter shows—with the dying child as the central actor, surrounded by people who know and love the child. And the younger the child, the less well we the community know the child; but we know the parents. We know their story. We understand their grief. Such grief is timeless, cross-cultural, and universal. Parents whose child has been diagnosed with a life-threatening illness, and especially parents whose child has died, feel as if they have lost part of themselves and lost it forever.

The death of a child is emotionally wrenching. A common feature of parental experience of a childhood death is a particular kind of grief, a unique kind of grief. This grief has been described by parents in many times and places. This poem by the eighth-century Chinese poet Bai Juyi illustrates feelings that are recognizable to parents in twenty-first-century America:

The sickness came, took only ten days,
even though we'd raised you for three years.
Miserable tears, crying voices, everything hurt painfully.
Your old clothes lonely on the hanger,
the medicine at your bedside.
I sent you through the deep village lanes,
I saw the tiny grave in the field.
Don't tell me it's three *li* away--
this separation is till the end of days.[15]

This is echoed in stories from other times and other places.

Linda McMahon analyzes a mother's account of her three-year-old son's death from smallpox, written in 1781. The mother, Lowry Wister, writes of her desperate efforts to cure her son of smallpox. The efforts were unsuccessful. She writes:

The (last) hours of his life were truly and sorrowfully painful to him and the reflections upon them at this day are so truly afflicting and distressing to me his sorrowing mother that I cannot commit them to writing. Oh! my son my son my dearly beloved child, thy pure spirit took its flight to the mansion of eternal glory to the habitations of never ending felicity, may God in his infinite mercy grant us an admittance into the same happy regions may we be again united is the fervent prayer of my afflicted soul in thy own time Lord Jesus grant it.[16]

"While eighteenth-century conventions stressed quiet resignation to God's will," McMahon concludes, "emerging cultural changes increasingly enabled—indeed, encouraged—women to give public voice to their private emotions. Individual women challenged cultural norms and helped usher in new forms of emotional and literary expression."[17]

One of the most famously public examples of such emotional trauma was Mary Todd Lincoln's response to the death of her twelve-year-old son Willie. After Willie's death, Mrs. Lincoln had a nervous breakdown and began to suffer from severe depression. She sought solace by consulting mediums who promised contact with her dead son. She even held a séance in the White House. These expressions of grief are mirrored by more recent parental narratives. Vicki Forman, writing about the death of her premature baby, describes her feelings:

I learned about grief during this time. I learned that no matter the true temperature, grief made the air crisp and cold; that it caused me to drive slowly, carefully; there was very little I could eat. The world receded. Everything took place in slow motion and was viewed as if down a very long telescope. So much was unfamiliar that if asked my name, I had to think for long moments. Grief is a visceral process.[18]

Amy Kuebelbeck has written about what it was like to receive a prenatal diagnosis of hypoplastic left heart syndrome, a congenital anomaly for which surgery is sometimes successful but from which many babies die in spite of surgery.[19] The Kuebelbeck family decided that they didn't want to put their baby, Gabriel, through surgery. And they didn't want to terminate the pregnancy either. She writes about what it was like to get the terrible diagnosis: "People often use physical terms to try to describe what it feels like to hear devastating news—that it's like being punched in the stomach, like being hit by a truck, or like the world is crashing in on them. To me it felt like falling backward, as though the tiled concrete floor, the clay underground, all the subterranean layers of rock were simply and soundlessly parting to let me through to some other dimension." But she also talks about some of the specialness of existing in the living-dying interval as she and her family waited for Gabriel to be born, knowing that he would die:

What followed was an extraordinary journey of grief, joy and love as we waited with Gabriel, simultaneously preparing for our son's birth and for his death. Despite some wrenchingly aggressive surgical options, no one could give our son a good heart. So we set out to give him a good life … . The months of waiting culminated in two-and-a-half peaceful hours of cradling Gabriel in our arms, in the same bed where he was born, surrounded by family and friends until his imperfect little heart finally stopped beating altogether. As we had written in our birth plan, "Our overriding wish is that our son Gabriel's birth and short life be filled only with comfort and love." And it was.

Empirical Studies of Pediatric Palliative Care

We can also learn about childhood death from empirical studies of parental experiences as their children are dying. Such studies try to draw generalizable conclusions by looking for common themes among the reports of many different parents who have experienced the death of a child.

Empirical studies give important quantitative, standardized, and, thus, comparable data about the experiences of parents whose children are critically ill and dying. Because they start with a defined analytic framework, they are not open to the subjective experiences of the parents. They allow us to compare one parent's experience with that of another and to make generalizations about the ways that parents experience the deaths of children, the ways that doctors and nurses might improve their care for dying children, and in some cases, give hints about the experiences of the children themselves.

One of the first empirical studies to explore the quality of care for dying children was by Wolfe and colleagues who interviewed 103 parents of children who died of cancer between 1990 and 1997 at two Boston hospitals.[20] About half of the children died in the hospital and half of those were in the intensive care unit when they died. According to the parents, 89 percent of children experienced a lot or a great deal of suffering during the last month of life. Nevertheless, most parents were satisfied with the care that their children had received.

Hinds and colleagues interviewed 62 parents of children with cancer for whom conventional therapy had not led to control of the cancer.[21] The parents faced a decision about whether to enroll their children in phase I clinical trials of experimental drugs, whether to enroll their children in palliative care programs, or whether to continue treatment but limit it by agreeing to a do-not-resuscitate order. The interviews focused on the parents' conceptions of their role as a "good parent." The researchers found that parents had quite specific ideas of what they needed to do. Eight themes predominated: Good parents should do right by their child, be there for the child, convey love, set a good life example, advocate for their child, let the Lord lead, not allow suffering, and try to keep their child as healthy as is possible.

Renjilian and colleagues studied 69 parents and 45 children at the Children's Hospital of Philadelphia.[22] The researchers began with an observation from their clinical experience, namely, that "parents of children with life-threatening illnesses often use patterns of language (aphorisms, mantras, or maxims) in conversations about decision-making." They wanted to understand whether these patterns of language and thought, or "heuristics," helped parents make decisions. They give some examples; prototypical phrases that function as explicit heuristics might include "We will always choose the option that most improves her quality of life" and "We always said we would do anything to fight this disease." They found that parents do tend to focus on a phrase or two to describe their response to the clinical complexities of their child's situation. For example, the most common heuristics were "I want my child to be comfortable," "I want my child to have a quality of life," and "I don't want my child to be in pain." These were said by 42 percent, 39 percent, and 32 percent of parents respectively. Renjilian et al. suggest that these mottos or mantras "enable parents to make decisions with greater efficiency than deliberative decision-making models, focused on risks and benefits, pros or cons, or maximizing expected utility."

Overall, empirical studies show that well-organized pediatric palliative care programs can help parents find ways to make sense of complex information and help diagnose and treat symptoms, pain, and suffering in critically ill children. The studies also show gaps in the processes, misunderstandings about what children need, and missed opportunities to improve care.

One problem with most studies of pediatric palliative care is that they are retrospective studies performed after children have died.[23, 24, 25] This is understandable. It is also inevitably misleading because the decisions and conversations that take place in the ICU or the oncology ward often take place while the prognosis is uncertain. Some children die, others don't. Parents whose children were critically ill but didn't die probably have different views of the situations that they faced. Because the outcome was different, they probably come away from such experiences with very different attitudes and beliefs.

A common theme in studies of parents whose children died is that doctors gave them false hope or withheld information about how sick the child really was. By contrast, parents whose children were close to death but who survived are more likely to be angry at doctors for giving a bleak prognosis and taking away hope.[26, 27]

In addition to this selection bias in the studies, there is another problem with the existing literature. The studies are inevitably retrospective studies that rely on parents' recall of the events at the time of their child's death. But, as Meert and colleagues note, "Parents' perceptions and desires expressed after their child's death may or may not relate to their actual needs at the time of the death. Parents are often angry after their child's death; anger and blame directed at others may be a form of unresolved grief."[28]

Conclusion

Childhood death is different today than it has ever been in the past. It is rarer. It requires a different sort of parental involvement. It makes different demands on doctors and nurses. We have come to understand the experiences of life-threatening childhood illnesses through careful studies of parental perceptions and through personal narratives by parents about their experiences.

The way that we think about critically ill children and the way we care for them and their parents is important for those children and their parents and is central to any art of dying. It is also an important representation of societal values with regard to the most desperately suffering among us.

Kenzaburo Oe captures the duality of personal and universal suffering in his autobiographical novel about a father who is caring for his critically ill baby. At one point, the father is discussing the situation with a friend. He starts with a description of the same sort of isolation that Moore and Hemon describe. "It's entirely a personal matter," he says. "What I'm experiencing personally now is like digging a vertical mine shaft in isolation; it goes straight down to a hopeless depth and never opens on anybody else's world. So I can sweat and suffer in that same dark cave and my personal experience won't result in so much as a fragment of significance for anybody else."

But he doesn't quite believe it. He also recognizes that his experience, while unique, has elements of the universal. "With some personal experiences that lead you way into a cave all by yourself," he notes, "you must eventually come to a side tunnel or something that opens on a truth that concerns not just yourself but everyone."

Notes

1. Alexander Hemon, "The Aquarium: A Child's Isolating Illness," *The New Yorker*, June 13, 2011.

2. Lorrie Moore, "People Like That Are the Only People Here," in *Birds of America* (Picador, 1988), 215.

3. Louisa May Alcott, *Little Women Wedded* (Sampson Low, Marston, Low, & Searle, 1872), 174.

4. Source: http://charlesdickenspage.com/carol.html.

5. Source: http://www.poetryconnection.net/poets/Dylan_Thomas/1093.

6. Historical Ken, http://passionforthepast.blogspot.com/2011_07_01_archive.html, July 10, 2011, quoting Karen Rae Mehaffy's *Rachel Weeping: Mourning in 19th Century America*.

7. Katherine J. Gold, Vanessa K. Dalton, and Thomas L. Schwenk, "Hospital Care for Parents after Perinatal Death," *Obstetrics & Gynecology* 109, no. 5 (2007): 1156–1166.

8. "Stillbirth and neonatal death" (http://www.myjewishlearning.com/life/Life_Events/Death_and_Mourning/Contemporary_Issues/StillbirthNeonatal_Loss.shtml).

9. Sinclair Lewis, *Arrowsmith*, 1925 (Signet, 2008).

10. "Early Uses of Diphtheria Antitoxin in the United States" (http://www.historyof vaccines.org/content/blog/early-uses-diphtheria-antitoxin-united-states).

11. Mikhaíl Bulgakov, *A Country Doctor's Notebook*, tr. Michael Glenny (Melville House, 2013).

12. William Carlos Williams, *The Doctor Stories* (New Directions, 1984).

13. Barbara M. Sourkes, *The Deepening Shade: Psychological Aspects of Life-Threatening Illness* (University of Pittsburgh Press, 1982), 55.

14. Elisabeth Kübler-Ross, *On Death and Dying* (Scribner, 1997), 36.

15. "This parting is for all time" (http://www.consolatio.com/2007/09/bai-juyi-this -p.html).

16. Lowry Wister, "The Narrative of My Dearly Beloved Child," in Lucia McMahon, "So Truly Afflicting and Distressing to Me His Sorrowing Mother: Expressions of Maternal Grief in Eighteenth-Century Philadelphia," *Journal of the Early Republic* 32, no. 1 (2012): 27–60.

17. Ibid.

18. Vicki Forman, *This Lovely Life: A Memoir of Premature Motherhood* (Houghton Mifflin Harcourt, 2009), 1.

19. Amy Kuebelbeck, "Waiting with Gabriel," *Current Problems in Pediatric and Adolescent Health Care* 41, no. 4 (2011): 113–114.

20. Joanne Wolfe et al., "Symptoms and Suffering at the End of Life in Children with Cancer," *New England Journal of Medicine* 342, no. 5 (2000): 326–333.

21. Pamela S. Hinds et al., "Trying to be a Good Parent as Defined by Interviews with Parents who Made Phase I, Terminal Care, and Resuscitation Decisions for their Children," *Journal of Clinical Oncology* 27, no. 35 (2009): 5979–5985.

22. Chris B. Renjilian et al., "Parental Explicit Heuristics in Decision-Making for Children with Life-Threatening Illnesses," *Pediatrics* 131, no. 2 (2013): e566–e572.

23. Kathleen L. Meert et al., "Parents' Perspectives on Physician-Parent Communication Near the Time of a Child's Death in the Pediatric Intensive Care Unit," *Pediatric Critical Care Medicine* 9, no. 1 (2008): 2–7.

24. Elaine C. Meyer et al., "Improving the Quality of End-of-Life Care in the Pediatric Intensive Care Unit: Parents' Priorities and Recommendations," *Pediatrics* 117 (2006): 649–657.

25. Kelly N. Michelson, Linda Emanuel, et al., "Pediatric Intensive Care Unit Family Conferences: One Mode of Communication for Discussing End-of-Life Care Decisions," *Pediatric Critical Care Medicine* 12 (2011): e336–e343.

26. Tanis Miller, "Shalebug," *Current Problems in Pediatric and Adolescent Health Care* 41 (2011): 121–123.

27. Kelley Benham French, "Never Let Go," *Tampa Bay Times*, December 6, 2012.

28. Meert et al., "Parents' Perspectives on Physician-Parent Communication Near the Time of a Child's Death in the Pediatric Intensive Care Unit."

9   The Elderly and Dementia

Daniel Callahan

Not long ago I read a gripping but also wrenching book by a pediatrician on the care of dying children. I could hardly stand to read it, but I couldn't put it down. What can be worse than the death of a child, especially now that such deaths are comparatively rare? But as I became engrossed in the problem of caring for those at the opposite end of life, those with Alzheimer's Disease, I came to think that a family member caring for a spouse or parent with the disease may have an almost equally heavy, if much different, burden to bear. The dying elderly can require care for much longer, and the difficulty of care rises as the disease progresses, an altogether unpleasant and demanding situation. But if death in childhood is rare and still declining, the prevalence of Alzheimer's Disease is headed in the opposite direction, with a parallel increase in the number of distressed caretakers at the family level and at the institutional level.

A glance at the scope of Alzheimer's Disease tells its national story, which is profoundly disturbing. One eighth of those over the age of 65 in the United States now have Alzheimer's Disease, and it is the sixth leading cause of death. In 2010, there were 454,000 new diagnoses, and that number is projected to increase to 615,000 in 2030 and to nearly a million in 2050. The total number of seniors over age 65 with Alzheimer's Disease in 2050 is expected to be between 11 million and 16 million. Two hundred billion dollars were spent on treating Alzheimer's in 2012, and that is expected to increase to a trillion in 2050. There are now about 15 million unpaid caretakers. Few of them will avoid grief to a larger or smaller degree; grief appears as a predictable, almost inherent part of providing lengthy, demanding care.

There is now a large and illuminating research literature on grief and Alzheimer's Disease, and I will briefly summarize its findings. I will do so in order to set the stage for a discussion of the moral problems facing individual caretakers and the stress they experience while managing the physical dying of their loved ones. I will then address the larger social problem of intergenerational responsibility: what do the young owe the old when the latter are sick and dying?

A comparison comes to mind, at the other end of the age spectrum. There are, it is estimated, about 6 million grandparents caring for their grandchildren, many of whom didn't bargain for that responsibility when they become parents themselves. So too with Alzheimer's Disease: as children grow up, and even into adulthood, they didn't bargain for being forced into the caretaker role when their parents became old. Nor when people marry do most bargain for the reality of "in sickness and in health" when it encompasses years of care for a person who is not only physically dying but whose selfhood has died before his or her bodily death. The grief that double death engenders, if not utterly unique in medicine, is at once common and predictable while also painfully unique, with a wide range of responses among individual Alzheimer's caretakers.

Tolstoy famously wrote that "all happy families are alike; each unhappy family is unhappy in its own way." It can no less be said of the grief of caretakers that they are all perhaps more alike when the person cared for is doing well early on, but each is different when confronted with stark displays of the cognitive decay and destruction of a person they once knew as intact and competent.

The Breadth and Depth of Caretakers' Burdens

Variation in caretakers' responses is important to keep in mind, primarily because there exist any number of ways to respond to the many manifestations of grief. A sense of sadness and loss is pervasive, but so are many things. They include the decline of ordinary social interactions outside of the demanding role of caretaker, caught very acutely in the title of a 1981 book, *36 Hour Day;* the strain on the health, physical and mental, of the caretaker; the loss of a job or occupation while providing the care; the diminishment of control of one's life, stolen away by care for someone whose life has already been filched by the disease; guilt and moral ambiguity; a decline in outside recreational activities; the loss of previously established marital or filial roles (the child of the parent forced to reverse family roles); the length of time of the disease, which can stretch into many years; anger, fatigue, frustration, regret; the often different kinds of grief and response shaped by home care or institutionalization; the recognition that the future of the care is likely to be more demanding than the present situation but no less certain to turn out poorly; and the loss of intimacy and emotional relationship with a person who is no longer the same person with whom the caregiver once had that connection—a person who has died in every way save for his or her enduring body.[1]

That is a dizzying array of symptoms, perhaps matched in part by the care of those with other diseases, though other chronic illnesses rarely necessitate the kind of long-term intensity required of the Alzheimer's caretaker. Those who provide care for the elderly with dementia observe the decline and loss of the personhood of the one cared for, and, at the same time, remain all too aware that their own personhood is being severely damaged in the process, ground down by the unrelenting nature of the disease.

One quotation in the grief literature particularly caught my eye, capturing the sense of caretaker oppression:

The hardest part of all this is watching a loved one die a little each day. My mother was so smart, skipping two grades in school and what an excellent memory. What went wrong? People say it is hard to watch a person die of cancer. Well, now I have seen a dad die of cancer and a mother slowly die of Alzheimer's Disease. I would take cancer any day of the week. There are services to help families deal with the grief after a loved one dies of cancer. What services are there for my grief? Just a person to say 'well things are only going to get worse.' My grief is nowhere near being dealt with. I still have at least 5 more years of having no grief support.[2]

For a variety of reasons, a minority of caregivers report no grief.[3] For some, there remains some degree of intimacy and a capacity also to focus attention on what relationship still remains, not on the downhill future. The religious beliefs of others allow a certain equanimity. For still others, the lack of a strong earlier relationship tends to deaden a grief response. They are in a sense uncaring caretakers, motivated by duty, not affection, but quite capable of anger at their situation, all too aware of what they have had to sacrifice in their own lives, so much not chosen, too much unsought. For some as well, however, their caretaking was judged by them to have promoted their personal growth, defined as "a process of becoming more caring and connected to others, evaluating what is really meaning in life, and reassigning priorities."[4] Some researchers report that between 55 percent and 90 percent of all caretakers cite that as a feature of their other-wise overburdened life.[5]

The Paradox of Guilt

If there seems to be a paradox in that last finding, it is matched by the report of guilt as a common problem. The paradox, or so it appears to me, is that a feature of much of the moral life of people is a mix of well-deserved guilt for a failure to live up to some ethical ideals or values with a some-times equally strong sense of guilt, even when the right thing has been done and no guilt should be felt. No doubt there are some caretakers who are insensitive, careless and lazy in the care they provide, but many more I would guess fall into the latter group. Four types of guilt among caretakers appear to be common:

• the guilt occasioned by anger that is not fully repressed toward the patient, either because of abusive language and hostile or embarrassing behavior, or simply because of the burden of care itself and the challenge it poses to one's freedom and independence

• guilt because the care never seems to be enough, however hard one tries and however actually satisfactory and optimal the care

• the guilt from institutionalizing someone even when it will serve the patient better and be a perfectly reasonable way of relieving some of the caretaker burden

• wishing the death of the patient, particularly when his selfhood has clearly been destroyed and no communication or self-care is any longer possible. Her life has come to an end, but why then is she still living on?

Why do caretakers feel guilty and often berate themselves for doing so, particularly when they and others believe it to be the good, humane, car-ing thing to do? That can seem strange and inexplicable, out of line with other more understandable range of common troubling emotions. Though it may seem something of a stretch to suggest that there is a single explana-tion for all these manifestations of guilt, or only a few, I want to suggest five possible sources of guilt:

• a caretaker's occasional temptation to do the wrong thing, or to pass unworthy, unfair judgments—judgments that lurk just below the surface even if never acted upon (like the biblical condemnation of adultery in one's heart, even if not in one's marital behavior)

• the sense that an undeserved, unlucky, and inexplicable fate has befallen the caretaker

• doing the right thing for someone when it is personally beneficial to the caretaker, with tension between a rational decision to institutionalize a patient and a desire not to do so because of self-interest—an example of making a rational decision, and one so recognized by others, yet with a lurking suspicion nonetheless that the "real" motive is less worthy of praise

• the psychological and moral dilemma of wishing for something generally judged to be wrong, but perhaps a common desire: hoping that the patient with advanced Alzheimer's Disease will die, but understanding that common morality doesn't allow that kind of wish

• the fact that the ethical standards for the extent and limits of children's obligations to their parents or a spouse aren't clear.

Moral Obligations of Children and Parents

In what follows, I will pursue only the problem of the obligations of children to elderly parents and of spouses to care for each other. Marriage these days bears a confused status: how many spouses still promise to care for each other "for better or worse, in sickness and in health?" I have no idea, and probably no one does, but I believe there is still an implicit agreement that they will care for each other in those ways. At the least there would be some, and maybe considerable, condemnation of a spouse who simply abandons outright a spouse who contracted Alzheimer's Disease (though I have no doubt it happens). But if in the past—as when the *Ars moriendi* was at its prime—caring for a spouse sick from most diseases was usually a short-term job. Alzheimer's Disease has brought a radical change. The disease often stretches out for many years, often long enough to wreak havoc not only on the health of the caretaker and social life of the spouse but also on the spouses' relationship, destroying it altogether at the end. That is a heavy demand, more than many people can endure. Are there some limits, some point at which a spouse could be released from that burden? If so, they are wholly unwritten and thus vague.

But it wouldn't seem wrong for a spouse enduring the unendurable to institutionalize the other spouse, particularly if there was no reason to believe that the institutionalized spouse would be made worse off. It might seem more altruistic to continue the home care, but it is hard to see how institutionalizing someone could be considered morally wrong. That the spouse might once have earlier said that he didn't want to be taken out of the home doesn't seem a compelling reason not to do so—particularly in the advanced stages of the illness, where cognition and human interactions have all but disappeared. The grief literature makes clear, however, that the burden of guilt is much less for children who institutionalize parents than for spouses when they do so.[6] The former have had a burden lifted from them while the latter may be more torn with doubt (and often compensating by constant, even excessive visits and monitoring of care).

If the obligations of spouses to care for each other—shaped by some informal norms that impose a duty to care, and with personal costs—are marked by uncertainty about its range and limits, the obligation of children to care for parents is no less ambiguous. Historically, it was long understood that children had a strong obligation to care for their parents, and that the family was the main foundation for that duty. Though there are stories of Eskimos' putting their elderly on ice floes as a way of ridding themselves of an economic burden in the face of serious food shortages, that was probably uncommon. The elderly of earlier generations didn't generally live long lives, much less with the multiple chronic illnesses that now mark their lives. Even if feeble, they could perform modest work compatible with their strength. There was no such thing as retirement, only a gradually reduced set of duties.

Legal Demands and Changing Social Practices

By the nineteenth century, and no doubt with the advent of industrialization, more formal moral duties were developed, legally requiring financial support of the aged by their children. Behind that change was a well-articulated principle of reciprocity: just as parents had taken care of their dependent children so also those children should care for their parents when they became unable to care for themselves. The English legal scholar William Blackstone articulated that view well in his *Commentaries*: "The duties of children to their parents arise from a principle of natural justice and retribution. For to those who gave us existence we naturally owe subjection and obedience during our minority, and honor and reverence thereafter; they who protected the weakness of our infancy are entitled to our protection in the infirmity of their age."[7]

There have been many objections to the supposed moral symmetry of the parent-child relationship, but nonetheless it endured and led to two later developments. One was the emergence of the English "poor laws" designed in part to relive the burden of parent care on children, and the precursor of twentieth-century social policies designed to shift the burden from family care of the old to government support. The other was the adoption of many laws at the state level in the United States establishing a legal requirement that children support their parents when the parents could no longer support themselves. But Medicare and Social Security made those laws less necessary, and public opinion polls indicated a declining belief on the part of the public of children's duty to care for elderly parents. The laws were gradually taken off the books in the course of the twentieth century.

Nonetheless, despite the gradual disappearance (or non-enforcement) of legal obligations to provide care, and despite the emergence of government programs, I believe that the concept of a duty of children to care for elderly parents is alive and well. For one thing, the government programs by no means provide full financial support, especially for long-term nursing care. Save for the affluent elderly with good pension support from their earlier work life, or from their savings, the majority requires some help. No less important, parent-child relationships marked by love and affection, and stimulated by the physical and other decline brought on by aging in general, inspire a desire to help parents. The thousands of daughters (or less commonly sons) who make enormous sacrifices of their own lives and time, and show willingness to put up with considerable travail of various other kinds, provide good evidence of a willingness to care that is not socially or legally required in any formal sense.

To go the second mile, whether out of some sense of duty, or altruism, or pity, is admirable. These adult children could run away, but they choose to stay. They could institutionalize their parents, but even in the face of common sense, or stimulated by guilt, they honor the earlier spoken desire of a parent not to have that done. In all of the research literature on Alzheimer's care, I have not seen a rich analysis of what motivates caretakers to give up so much of their own lives to care for another. It seems almost identical to the way parents will make no end of sacrifices to care for a sick or dying child. Human nature has its good side.

End-of-Life Care

My wife is the legal guardian of her demented 99-year-old stepmother, cared for in an institution artfully described as a home for the memory-impaired. My wife is lucky: the stepmother was married to a wealthy man whose will left her with enough money to pay the $135,000 annual cost of her care (not to mention many side costs). She has been in that institution more than ten years, gradually losing her ability to recognize others, to talk, to feed herself or have any interaction with others. She is dead, so to speak, as a person, but she is alive in her body, with no imminent threats to her survival. She left behind her advance directives not to receive life-extending medical treatment of any kind, and her institution has been instructed not to call EMS if a medical problem appears. This is a common situation now, a tribute one might say to the power of modern medicine to extend life, but not much of a life at the age of 99 with advanced Alzheimer's Disease. But, save for euthanasia, which many others and I reject, she will live on for an indeterminate period. She is at one end of the spectrum.

At the other end are people in their eighties and their nineties with Alzheimer's Disease but suffering from multiple other chronic diseases (co-morbidities), any one of which has a possibility of killing them before Alzheimer's does. In those cases, decisions must be made to deal or not to deal with the co-morbidities, where more ordinary standards for end-of-life care can come into play. But should there be different, special ethical standards for treating the co-morbidities of those with Alzheimer's? My general answer would be No for those in the early and middle stages of the disease, where there is still some self-awareness, interaction with others, and reasonable expectations for beneficial treatment and possibly a few more years of life before the end stage. They still have a selfhood, diminished surely but not extinguished.

The last stage seems to me the one where the decision will be the most difficult. Let us assume that the self has been destroyed, that the patient has decisively moved out of the social and familial world, the past and present obliterated with nothing left but the death of the body as his future. If the patient has left an advance directive of the total kind—that is, under no circumstances should there be any kind of medical intervention at all at the onset of a crisis—then it should be honored and the patient allowed to die from any threatening co-morbidity. In that sense the Alzheimer's patient is treated like any other patient with a critical condition, who has a similar right to be spared an intervention.

Standards for End-of-Life Care and Co-Morbidities

What if there is a co-morbidity of a potentially fatal kind and there is neither an advance directive nor an appointed surrogate (the latter being the more likely in view of the estimate that not many more than 25 percent of patients have an advance directive)? For families asked to make final decisions, or physicians in cases where there are no family members at hand, guilt can easily make its appearance: many if not most of them probably will be glad to see their care burden come to an end and, in a common phrase, see the death as a "blessing." But as noted earlier, there can be ambivalence about feeling that way, in effect feeling guilty for having such thoughts. We are not supposed to wish the death of another, and particularly when it could medically be extended.

It may simply be impossible to avoid all guilt. Life is full of ways to make us feel guilty when there is no culpability at all; the driver, for instance, who unavoidably kills a child who has darted out into the street is never likely to feel totally blameless. But if perhaps guilt is unavoidable for some when a family agrees to stop treatment of a severely demented person, a rational case can nonetheless be made that it is the right thing to do.

I offer two principles. First, *no one should be forced to live longer now in the advanced stages of Alzheimer's Disease than she would have in a pre-technological era*. I believe that most people in earlier times, even as long ago as 40 or 50 years, counted it a "blessing" when such a person died. Medical interventions offered no benefit in such cases at all, and the mere extension of the bodily life of someone whose selfhood had disappeared couldn't be considered a human good. As has been shown throughout this volume, only the advent of an aggressive technological era, beginning in the 1950s and the 1960s, made a difference, shifting the balance from a bias toward non-treatment to one of treatment and the dominance of the technological imperative: if a patient can be treated with a technology, he should be treated. This bias is still powerful and with it a twin brother: when in doubt, it is better to treat than not to treat. With the severely demented patient, the rule should be: when in doubt, do not treat. Nothing good will be gained.

Second, *there is as great an obligation to prevent a lingering or painful death as to promote health and life.* Many, if not most, of the interventions to treat chronic illness carry with them some risk of pain and discomfort. Even if Alzheimer's patients in the end stage of the disease have lost a sense of self, they don't lose the capacity to feel pain and discomfort, and that can be observed from many facial and other bodily expressions. Why should they have to run any risk of that possibility knowing that, even if the intervention is medically successful, the patient has no meaningful life as a human being left, more of the meaningless same? A treatment that provides an immediate benefit of some kind *may* only set the patient up for a worse death in the future and should not be considered a value for a patient; and "may"—even as only a possibility—is a good enough reason not to intervene.[8]

The Future of Care for Those with Alzheimer's Disease

Thus far I have not touched on some of the important social policy issues pertinent to the care of Alzheimer's Disease. I will conclude the chapter with a few thoughts on those issues, none of which necessarily paint a happy scenario for the future. They fall into the muddle-through kind, trying to do the best we can in a difficult situation. But then Alzheimer's is a unique disease, and so is the unique situation of caregivers. Our society has never confronted a comparable situation, and it isn't yet clear how it will be managed in the future, or how well.

I offer first a utopian vision of an overall policy solution, one that takes into account the needs of the Alzheimer's patients and caretakers. The obvious need is for the Medicare and Medicaid programs to remain strong and robust and the Social Security system as well. The average Medicare recipient spends somewhere between $3,000 and $5,000 a year for out-of-pocket expenses. Those expenses must be paid from a combination of their Social Security income and whatever other income they may have from pension plans and private savings. The sad fact of the matter, however, is that some 40 percent of retirees will fall short of having enough retirement income, and for many more it will be a chronic struggle. Utopian Idea Number One is to have a unified health and economic program that covers well their health and economic security needs.

Utopian Idea Number Two pertains to caretakers whose burden is great. We must determine how to relieve some of that burden. That might mean financial support for unpaid caretakers even if not for 24-hours-a-day help, at least for a good portion of it. Moreover, it would be important to have Medicare coverage for counseling help for caretakers. Local communities would be given support for programs for the demented.

But reality must come to bear here. It is hard even to imagine what the cost would be for either Number One or Number Two, much less both at the same time. As has already been mentioned, there are 15 million mainly unpaid caretakers—and they may each need help for five to ten years; and of course that 15 million will increase rapidly in the future as the baby boomers retire. Run the numbers on the utopian ideas—no, maybe that wouldn't be a good idea; it might be conducive to cardiac arrest and general hysteria. Moreover, from a government and congressional perspective, unpaid caretakers are the ideal solution. Though often suffering and stressed, they are free. An interesting speculative question is whether the children of the retirees would be willing to see their Medicare withholding taxes raised to stratospheric heights to come anywhere near the utopian dreams. I doubt it.

I think the best that can be hoped for would be some government support of family caretakers based on income levels, and then for part-time relief only. As Ridenour and Cahill have also shown in this volume, the development of local efforts based on bonds of community is a more likely path. Neighbor will have to help neighbor, volunteers to provide respite breaks for caretakers, and local communities to provide occasions for counseling. If ever there was a call for grassroots initiatives, this is it.

Notes

1. I have found the following helpful for a more detailed explanation of this point: *Dementia and Aging: Ethics, Values, and Policy Choices*, ed. Robert H. Binstock, Stephen G. Post, and Peter J. Whitehouse (Johns Hopkins University Press, 1992); Richard A. Brumback, "Neuro-Pathology and Symptomatology in Alzheimer Disease: Implications for Caregiving and Competence," in *Ethical Foundations of Palliative Care for Alzheimer Disease*, ed. Ruth B. Purtilo and Henk A. ten Have (Johns Hopkins University Press, 2004), 24–46; Cynthia Loos and Alan Bowd, "Caregivers of Persons with Alzheimer's Disease: Some Neglected Implications," *Death Studies* 21 (1992):

501–514; Kenneth L. Doka, ed., *Alzheimer's Disease: Living with Grief* (Hospice Foundation of America, 2004); Richard L. O'Brien, "Darkness Cometh: Personal, Social and Economic Burdens of Alzheimer Disease; Richard A. Brumback, "Neuro-Pathology and Symptomatology in Alzheimer Disease," in *Ethical Foundations*, ed. Purtillo and ten Have, 24–46; Kenneth K. Doka, ed., *Alzheimer's Disease: Living with Grief* (Hospice Foundation of America, 2004); Samuel J. Marwit and Robert M. Meuser, "Development and Initial Validation of an Inventory to Assess Grief in Caregivers of Persons with Alzheimer Disease." *The Gerontologist* 42 (2009): 756–765; Carol H. Ott, Sara Sanders, and Sheryl T. Kelber, "Grief and Personal Growth Experience of Spouses and Adult-Child Caregivers of Individuals with Alzheimer's Disease and Related Dementias," *The Gerontologist* 47 (2007): 798–807; Sara Sanders and Constance Corley, "Are They Grieving? A Qualitative Analysis Examining Grief in Caretakers of Individuals with Alzheimer's Disease," *Social Work in Health Care* 37 (2003): 35–53; Judah L. Ronch, "Mourning and Grief in Later Life Alzheimer's Dementia: Revisiting The Vanishing Self," *American Journal of Alzheimer's Disease* (1996): 25–28; Sara Sanders et al., "The Experience of High Levels of Grief in Persons with Alzheimer's Disease and Related Dementia," *Death Studies* 32 (2008): 495–523.

2. Sanders and Corley, "Are They Grieving?" 49.

3. Ott, "Grief and Personal Growth Experience," 789.

4. Ibid., 799.

5. Marwit and Meuser, "Development and Initial Validation of an Inventory," 751.

6. Ibid., 760.

7. Cited in Daniel Callahan, "Terminating Life-Sustaining Treatment for the Demented," *Hastings Center Report* 25 (1995): 88.

8. Callahan develops these principles more fully in "Terminating Life-Sustaining Treatment."

10 AIDS, the Modern Plague

Peter A. Selwyn

Thirty years have passed since the onslaught of the AIDS epidemic in the United States, a generation-long time period that has seen profound changes in how people with AIDS live and die. At first AIDS was a mysterious and terrifying plague; then it was a more narrowly circumscribed, medically manageable disease. Its fundamental clinical characteristics as an illness were completely transformed in little more than ten years. Most recently, for long-term survivors first infected in the 1980s, the disease has become a complex mix of multiple co-morbidities and "accelerated aging" over a much longer trajectory; patients pass through life milestones that they had never thought they would reach, accumulating more and more co-morbid illnesses along the way. These include conditions such as heart disease, diabetes, kidney or liver failure, osteoporosis, neurodegenerative disease, and a range of cancers that are not specific to AIDS or its causative virus, HIV. The irony, not lost on some, is that the "success" of surviving longer with HIV now brings with it the "reward" of being vulnerable to illnesses that, in an earlier era, those infected with HIV wouldn't have lived long enough to experience. During this evolution, AIDS has both shaped and reflected how we think about the dying process and death itself. Lessons from the care of patients dying from AIDS offer illustrations that hint toward what might be a contemporary *Ars moriendi* or art of dying.

Early AIDS as Plague: Stepping Into the Waves

In the early 1980s, after a long postwar period of advances in medical therapeutics that has been termed the *pax antibiotica*,[1] AIDS emerged as if from nowhere. It was a rapidly fatal illness that killed young adults with brutal efficiency, a plague with which modern society had no experience. Not only were these young men, women, and sometimes even children dying before their expected time; they were dying of a wide array of infectious diseases and rare cancers that had never been seen in such concentrations in any one population. The disease progressed fiercely and relentlessly, and doctors often had no choice but to observe helplessly as the common complicating milestones—oral thrush, bacterial pneumonia, *pneumocystis carinii* pneumonia, cerebral toxoplasmosis, cryptococcal meningitis, disseminated *m. avium complex* disease—flashed by like the stations left behind by a runaway train. We learned over time to diagnose and treat these complications better, and eventually to prevent some of them, but for close to a decade there was little if anything we could do to change the speed or the direction of the train.

This was a time of vulnerability for both patients and their care providers, and also a time of solidarity; there was a palpable sense that everyone was in it together. Both patients and clinicians felt the absence of the protective medical armamentarium upon which physicians rely in order to shield themselves from feeling helpless. So we doctors from the early years of AIDS learned simply to be present. Out of our medical comfort zone where doctors are accustomed to trying to isolate and fix specific problems, we learned the power of empathic listening, witnessing, and accompanying patients and families along this difficult journey. I had a social work colleague from those years who would describe the feeling of "stepping into the waves," to take the hand of each new patient who was washing up onto the beach. She knew that each one needed her as much as the last one she had gone to help out of the water, and that there would be an endless number of new ones to take their places, but the act of reaching out, of comforting, of accompanying, was the same for each.

Without the familiar tools that serve to routinize our interactions with patients and give the perception (if not illusion) of control over life and death—antibiotics, chemotherapy, surgery—we learned by necessity of the importance of being with patients, without turning away, through the course of a fatal disease. It took a disease we couldn't cure to teach us the true meaning of healing.

With no treatment even imaginable, and before the fundamental pathogenesis of AIDS as a blood-borne, virally transmitted illness had even been envisioned, we faced much fear, ignorance, and associated stigma. This wasn't yet the stuff of celebrity benefit concerts or fundraising walks; it was too raw, too dreadful, too untamed. Any association with AIDS tended to engender stigma, discomfort, and a sense of the dangerous "other." This social distancing extended both to patients and to their care providers; people with AIDS were routinely shunned, dismissed from jobs, blamed for having "brought this on" themselves, or declared to be receiving God's punishment for their immoral behavior. As a doctor, I experienced more subtle social distancing: after learning at a cocktail party of my occupation, a new acquaintance would make a discreet trip to the bathroom in order to wash his hands.

Yet this type of exclusion also united patients and their caregivers as part of a special community of loss and suffering. Rejected or ignored by the rest of society, which was initially quite slow to respond to the disease even at the highest levels of government, many of those affected by AIDS created social networks of caring and support, both within and outside of traditional medical systems. By the mid 1980s, in the most geographically concentrated areas—starting in urban New York and California—the disease had begun to affect multiple members of high-risk populations in a manner that escalated dramatically. Before long, in those early years, everyone in certain affected communities knew someone who had AIDS or who had died of it. Social networks began to be infiltrated by disease, first as isolated cases, and then in a growing swell of commonality. This pattern would repeat itself in villages in sub-Saharan Africa more than a decade later, where coffin makers began to observe an inexorable and unprecedented increase in demand for their craft as the epidemic spread. The disease continued to take hold, and the number of funerals in certain urban neighborhoods in New York and California began to grow eerily beyond anyone's expectations.

Multiple losses led both to a greater burden on the affected communities and to a sense of shared loss and solidarity in suffering that was less isolating than for those who perceived themselves to be suffering alone. Such solidarity in suffering also led to memorable acts of courage, and sacrifice, such as when ACT-UP activists chained themselves to the gates of the National Institutes of Health demanding increased access to experimental therapies. On another occasion, during the first placebo-controlled trial of AZT (also called zidovudine)—the first and only antiretroviral agent available at the time—study participants defied the study investigators and decided to mix the placebo pills with the active drug pills. Each would then draw from the combined pool in order that everyone would be able to have at least some of the active drug. In many instances, infected partners at different stages of advanced HIV disease continued lovingly to care for each other even as the disease threatened their physical and mental faculties. In many ways, just as it carried stigma and opprobrium in the larger society, AIDS brought out the brave and shining humanity of many of those personally affected by it.

I recall a couple of years later, after AZT had been approved and was in clinical use, being at a rally in Washington in support of more government funding for AIDS. In a sea of marchers I suddenly became aware of the repetitive sounds of beeper alarms and other electronic chirps rippling through the crowd: these were the every-four-hour alarms of patients who, at the time, had no choice but to take AZT six times per day. In those early days when AZT was the only available treatment, it came in high doses with severe side effects, and yet patients did whatever they could to make sure that they didn't miss a single dose.

Now the standard treatment for HIV infection is one pill once a day, combining three medications in one pill, with much greater efficacy and much less toxicity; the stakes seem somehow less dramatic, the act of taking daily medications more mundane. Much of the focus of clinical visits for patients with AIDS is now on "adherence," and the medical literature abounds with reports of different strategies to ensure adherence and help patients remember to take their daily doses; poor adherence is the leading cause of the development of HIV resistance. These concerns were not on the horizon in those early years, when even the act of prescribing AZT— toxic, not very effective, difficult to take—seemed like a sacrament.

The power of the affected community was palpable not only in the fierce desire to live and to provide support in surviving, but also in the experience of death. Mutual support in bereavement, the importance of group and community rituals, and the use of art and music as channels for remembrance, celebration, and transcendence, were all powerful counterpoints to the experience of medical helplessness in witnessing this spreading plague. Friends, family members, caregivers, and volunteers came together out of necessity, commitment, and love, with the basic dedication to ease the burden of suffering as the disease ravaged individuals, families, and communities.

For patients and populations that were too readily written off or marginalized by the mainstream, the simple act of memorializing took on great power and meaning. I recall going to a concert one evening at the Cathedral of St. John the Divine in New York City. It was some years into the epidemic, and I stopped in front of a simple candle-lit parchment on the wall of an alcove with the words written on it, "In memory of those who have died of AIDS." Reading those words filled me suddenly with sadness, but at the same time inspiration, and with a kaleidoscope of memories I reflected on all my patients who by that time had died. On another occasion, I went with my family to view the AIDS Memorial Quilt which had been unfurled on the National Mall in Washington. Stretching from the Washington Monument to the Capitol, these stitched-together panels each told a powerful story of individuality, community, and love, and together amounted to an incredible evocation of the interconnected souls of all those who had been brought together by AIDS. Other times, more simply, in our AIDS treatment program, we would gather periodically—patients, families, staff—light a candle, and read the names of the patients who had died in the last month, stopping after each name to let our collective memories come into the room and linger in the candlelight.

When I initially started caring for patients with AIDS in the early 1980s, my first job was as medical director of the substance abuse treatment program at Montefiore Hospital in the Bronx, the same hospital where I had just finished training. This program, which consisted of close to 1000 current or former injection drug users on methadone maintenance therapy, was a site for some of the earliest studies of AIDS and drug use. Soon after the HIV (or then HTLV-III) antibody test was developed which enabled us to detect HIV on routine laboratory testing, we conducted one of the first studies funded by the Centers for Disease Control (CDC) of the prevalence of HIV infection among drug injectors. We found to our alarm that close to 50 percent of the patients were already infected with HIV. With no treatment available (AZT was introduced in 1987), we tried to prepare ourselves and the patients for the reality that all those infected probably were going to get sick and die within the next several years. This was both a grim assessment and also, oddly, a source of connection and community: patient support groups, peer education and outreach initiatives, and advocates for expanding AIDS services united in a common cause, resulting in a form of empowerment within the larger context of a loss of control.

Feeling helpless in the face of looming death and wanting at least to acknowledge the impact of this plague on our community, I started to go to patients' funerals. I recall the first I attended at a small funeral home in the South Bronx. I entered the darkened room uncomfortably. The casket sat at one end, and people sat in rows of chairs facing it. I felt somehow that the family would be angry with me for coming since I had not been able to save their son. (I had not yet learned to appreciate the role of the physician as witness to and partner with dying patients; I had at that point only internalized the larger cultural stereotype of physician as rescuer or savior.) Instead of being angry, the family was deeply moved and grateful to see me, all standing up to surround me, give me hugs, thank me for taking care of him and for coming to pay my respects. Other times, I would go to patients' funerals along with other patients from the methadone program, themselves HIV-infected, struck by their courage and community as they honored their friends who had died, just as they knew that they themselves probably would soon be in the same situation. I recall one patient, tall and by then stick-thin from advanced AIDS, getting up with great effort from his chair in the funeral home where his friend lay in the open coffin in the front of the room (the body also clearly emaciated from the disease, seeming very small, laid out in the oversize suit that didn't come close to fitting anymore). Standing by the edge of the coffin, resting his hand on it, the dying paying respects to the dead, seeming to bridge a very narrow divide between this world and the next.

Caring for so many young patients who were dying—most of them in their early to mid thirties, many of them within five years of my own age at the time—I felt both a greater kinship and a greater vulnerability than in my previous experience in medical school and residency, when the patients I had cared for who died were very few and also mostly much older. I remember watching a young father have to say goodbye to his two small children, feeling powerless to do anything to prevent his death, and then going home to my own two small children safely tucked in their beds for the night. This pulled at my heart in ways I have not experienced before or since, and it made me better able to support this patient and many others as they confronted these terrible situations along the way. I learned the difference between pity and compassion, between sympathy and empathy: the important distinction between feeling sorry *for* someone and feeling sorry *with* someone.

I also learned how these feelings of loss and sadness, triggered by my experiences with dying patients opened the way for me to appreciate and grieve my own losses, losses of which I had not been fully aware, most important the sudden death of my own father when I was an infant.[2] This was perhaps the greatest gift of working with AIDS patients, both for myself personally and in my role as a physician: recognizing that we are all living and dying, we all suffer loss, and that keeping our heart open to feel and experience our own pain is a powerful way both to help heal ourselves and be a healer for others.

For too long, doctors have been taught (whether overtly or by role modeling and the unconscious culture of medicine) to suppress their emotions or identification with the patient, as if this threatens to compromise professionalism or cloud clinical judgment. Though it is essential for professional caregivers not to let their own emotional issues interfere with effective care of patients, I believe that it is equally important for caregivers to keep their hearts open, to recognize their own vulnerability, losses, and less-than-omnipotence. In these ways doctors can be truly present with patients and offer deeper healing. The losses that we experience ourselves, the different but common ways in which we are all "broken" by the world, prime us to be able to understand and appreciate the pain and loss of our patients. A heart that has been broken gains greater capacity to connect with the suffering other. We are not professional voyeurs; we are, more humbly, partners, fellow travelers. As Leonard Cohen put it in his song "Anthem," "There is a crack in everything / That's where the light gets in." AIDS cracked open the facade of complacency that protected us from our own vulnerability; it disrupted everything, and also allowed our common humanity to shine through.

People described the onset of the AIDS epidemic as an earthquake or tsunami, arriving suddenly, unexpectedly, and devastating everything in its wake. Doctors were faced with an almost existential choice: do I stay, leave, or run toward the devastation? As with any disaster response, the initial tool bags were make-shift. In heavily affected areas, primary care doctors, infectious disease specialists, oncologists, and substance abuse treatment providers, each had to respond uniquely to the consequences of the disease expressing itself in their specific populations. But there was no credentialing, professional certification, or textbook; models of care and caring were developed by those who were on the front lines when AIDS hit. For the first generation of AIDS care providers, expertise was simply the byproduct of experience. It would take a decade for younger trainees and students to commit to AIDS care as a potential career option. And with the first generation of AIDS doctors on its way to retirement, there are, thankfully, more of these reinforcements on the way.

But as often happens in the aftermath of a crisis, the critical lessons fade with time. We have perhaps lost the humbling immediacy of relationship with patients, relationships characterized by caring for those in front of you without flinching, while recognizing full well that you cannot prevent what is coming next. It is, of course, a great relief that we now have more treatment options, and the sense of fate and inevitability which permeated those years is no longer the norm. Still, our ability to move comfortably, or at least with more familiarity, in caring for patients with AIDS, seems to have taken us further from the dying and further away from being simply present with those who are dying.

From Certain Death to Chronic Disease

Now AIDS has become a treatable, manageable disease; it has, in effect, become "tamed," to appropriate the term suggested by Philippe Aries,[3] by which I mean that its manifestations have been well described and are often controllable, its expression is more circumscribed, its trajectory less unstoppable. It is only when we see a patient who has not been able to benefit from the current treatment paradigm—whether as a result of delayed diagnosis, or social or behavioral problems interfering with care, or of other disparities in treatment access and outcome that are heavily weighted toward poor and underserved populations—that we are reminded of the unmediated force of the disease in its untreated form.

Despite being "tamed," AIDS still poses many challenges, including how to handle a chronic illness with multiple co-morbidities, and how to age with (as opposed to how to die with) the disease. These challenges can be overlooked amid the busyness and demands of routine clinical care. Furthermore, many of the AIDS specialists who trained after the advent of highly active antiretroviral therapy don't have substantial experience in working with patients at the end of life. This may result in an inattention toward issues related to the dying process, and may limit a doctor's ability to accompany patients through these phases when they do occur, as they inevitably do for all of us.

AIDS care, at least in its medical aspects, is now largely defined by a treatment paradigm which seeks to engage and maintain patients on antiretroviral therapy (or, more specifically, "highly active antiretroviral therapy," universally referred to as HAART). These therapeutic agents have been developed and marketed with astonishing speed, from the first characterization of the human immunodeficiency virus (HIV) in the mid 1980s, to the development of therapeutic strategies for drug development and testing, to the marketing and widespread use of more than 25 anti-HIV drugs in less than 20 years. These drugs have completely transformed the clinical management of HIV disease and AIDS, and for patients who are diagnosed and started on treatment before they have already experienced severe immunodeficiency, the projected lifespan has started to approximate that of comparable individuals without HIV infection.

While these changes in treatment for HIV/AIDS have been a welcome advance for patients and their care providers, the discussion surrounding antiretroviral therapy has now become more narrowly focused on patients' adherence to these medications, management of side effects, and monitoring of associated laboratory tests. These approaches mirror much of the broader practice of medicine, which tends to be reductionist and "problem-oriented." The implicit assumption is that problems are best addressed by isolating them, identifying the working and non-working parts, and then intervening to "fix" what doesn't work. The current treatment era has brought HIV much more squarely into this cultural comfort zone. The examining room discourse typically relies on questions such as, "What are my numbers?' and doctors may likewise dwell on the mechanics of how patients are taking their pills every day. When patients don't take their medications regularly, or when there are other problems that interfere with their ability to care for themselves—such as mental health problems, substance use, homelessness, or coexisting medical problems—this can lead to frustration and sometimes disaffection on the part of the patient, the doctor, or both. I recall a particularly exasperating clinic visit with a patient who insisted that he was taking his medications despite significant laboratory evidence to the contrary. Whereas in the pre-HAART era it felt as if the doctor and the patient were allied against the disease, it now sometimes feels as if the doctor and the therapy are allied against the patient—an unfortunate by-product of the emergence of the therapeutic era for HIV/AIDS.

Another consequence of the emergence of the successful treatment era for HIV/AIDS is that the outcome following a diagnosis of AIDS no longer follows a uniform, inevitable path. What has been referred to as the "grim democratization of AIDS" in the pre-treatment era, when all patients seemed to die rapidly and predictably, has now been replaced by a regrettably familiar pattern such as is seen for most if not all other chronic diseases, in which social inequalities, poverty, and marginalization of vulnerable populations have emerged in the HAART era. The current therapeutic paradigm has rapidly shifted, with good reason, to a focus on engagement and adherence with effective antiretroviral therapy. In short, patients are no longer "supposed to" die. The effectiveness of therapy implies that a death due to AIDS must be an aberration, a failure, an isolated event. Far from the days of frequent funerals and memorial services, now when patients with AIDS die, at least in the developed world, the implication, whether stated or even perceived, is that this should have been preventable. This may tend to impose an added burden on patients, caregivers, and survivors: that earlier community of shared suffering and experience is often no longer present; it has been replaced by individual regret, second-guessing, and assigning blame. Before treatment existed, when death was inevitable and the trajectory was swift and uniform, it seemed almost that dying was a matter of "fate"—that is, something unavoidable, universal, and expected. Once effective disease-modifying treatments became available, "fate" was somehow transformed into "tragedy," a separation between what was happening and what might have been, a terrain of "what ifs," choices taken and not taken, and more a function of individual responsibility and agency.[4] This brought more of a quality of empowerment for patients, who now had more potential control over their destinies in the treatment era, but it also could bring a more isolating feeling of personal failure when patients died, for both patients and doctors.

With less focus now on end-of-life issues in the daily experience of HIV/AIDS, death can be an uncomfortable and unwelcomed topic for physicians, patients, and families. This is particularly true for newer generations of AIDS care providers who didn't live through those early years when death was, unfortunately, not a stranger to anyone. As with other chronic illnesses such as diabetes, cardiovascular, or chronic pulmonary disease, clinicians often don't dwell on end-of-life care or the anticipation of death. Rather, they pay more attention to treating the acute complications and monitoring the exacerbations and remissions of a slowly progressive illness. While important, this focus also can obscure a more fundamental attention to the dynamics of disease progression, and the importance of addressing goals of care, anticipatory grief and loss, and other equally important issues that may not be as starkly defined as they once were. As a culture, and as a profession, we tend not to want to "go there." When the disease was untreatable, "going there" was unavoidable; now, as a profession, we are more comfortable surrounding ourselves and our patients with all the other more familiar comforts that compete for our attention.

Living and Dying with a View onto an Unfamiliar Landscape

Though no one would want to return to the terrible early years of the AIDS epidemic, I would hope that some of the lessons learned from that experience could continue to inform our current practice and sensibility. It was as if a window briefly opened onto a landscape unfamiliar to most physicians, in which we couldn't make use of many of the disease-modifying tools that had come to define late-twentieth-century medicine. Yet in that same landscape we could experience both the vulnerability and the power of accompanying our patients on the journey of dying, could learn how to witness and to be present for our patients and their families with an open heart, and could learn how to bring our own wounded humanity into this relationship without losing ourselves along the way. With the advent of the HAART era, that window has closed, and the day-to-day reality of medical care for AIDS has become much more narrowly defined. Combining effective disease treatment with the sensibility to move through to that other landscape remains a challenge.

Notes

1. Nicholas Wade, "Method and Madness: Pax Antibiotica," *New York Times*, October 15, 1995.

2. Peter A. Selwyn, *Surviving the Fall* (Yale University Press, 1998).

3. Philippe Ariès, *Western Attitudes toward Death: from the Middle Ages to the Present* (Johns Hopkins University Press, 1974).

4. Peter A. Selwyn and Robert Arnold, "From Fate to Tragedy: The Changing Meanings of Life, Death, and AIDS," *Annals of Internal Medicine* 129, no. 11 (1998): 899–902.

Conclusion: Toward a New Ethical Framework for the Art of Dying Well

Lydia S. Dugdale

The day I met Diana in the primary care clinic, I noticed that it took my medical assistant Jackie longer than usual to settle her in the examination room. When Jackie gave me the signal that Diana was ready, she whispered "There's a lot going on with her." I took a deep breath and braced myself; it was a Monday afternoon, I was running behind, and new patients with "a lot going on" typically don't help me get back on schedule.

I had hardly opened the door when a sophisticated, well-groomed woman in her mid sixties blurted out "I'm dying. I know I'm dying. I need you to help me through this." Diana hardly paused to inhale as she proceeded over the course of the next twenty minutes to tell me the story of her illness, of how just seven months earlier she had been the picture of health for a 66-year-old woman, of how in an instant she had found herself in the ICU on life support because of overwhelming sepsis, of how the doctors had found that the cause of the sepsis was a previously undiagnosed autoimmune condition run amok, of how she had been told that her disease was rapidly progressive and would soon be fatal, and of how she was "right this instant" making plans to hand over the reins of various academic projects she had been directing. After a split-second breath, during which I considered asking—on account of her unremitting speech—whether she had a history of overactive thyroid, she proceeded for another twenty minutes to deliver an account of her life story: of her grim upbringing, of her earlier failed marriage, of her current wonderful marriage, of those she considered her children, and of her various civic and professional involvements. All doctors know that there exists an art to interrupting the incessantly talking patient, and even though for the sake of my other waiting patients I should have plied that art, I did not; there is something sobering about meeting a self-consciously dying woman face-to-face and being asked to accompany her in her dying.

What struck me that day about Diana, and what approaches the heart of the *Ars moriendi*, was her firm and clear recognition of human finitude, her acknowledgment that life is bounded. How can we begin to describe a framework for an art of dying well if we don't first admit of limitation and death? We can't talk about the *art* of dying without first accepting that we will die. Art invites careful attention to the possibility of beauty and of flourishing. We must attend wisely to death; we must consider its excesses in light of its deprivation, its beauty in light of its decay. Only those who accept human mortality can experience an art of dying.

Diana further impressed me that day by the way in which her acknowledgment of finitude drove her to reflect on her life, which she largely summarized in reference to community. Community helps us to recognize frail hopes and joys that surface in the midst of adversity. Relationships clarify the goods that we value and the ends to which we orient ourselves. Having spent much of the past three years thinking about what might constitute a contemporary *Ars moriendi*, I conclude—at least provisionally—that an art of dying cannot develop without two central components: clear recognition of finitude and a strong sense of community. In the face of death, the calm acceptance of finitude and the embrace of community allows for flourishing even as the body fails.

Callahan's prescription for a peaceful death, which Lysaught describes in chapter 5, includes four components: acceptance by the patient, minimal pain, maximal consciousness, and the presence of community. While my provisional proposal for a contemporary art of dying appears to include only the first and last of these, sufficiently broad conceptions of finitude and community can include but also go far beyond the medical aspects of dying. A nuanced understanding of finitude by patient and physician, for example, attends to the effects of medical and technological developments. Physicians who seek to honor their dying patients' finitude necessarily aim to minimize their suffering; and in seeking to honor the patients' communities, they necessarily strive to maximize their patients' consciousness. Comprehensive conceptions of finitude and community—as I will show— can also address many other aspects of dying, including the spiritual, the secular, the personal, and the political.

Since the goal of this volume is to articulate a bioethical framework for dying well, we must ask in this final chapter whether we still hold that bioethics is well matched to the task. Concluding that only a broad conception of bioethics can encourage both the contemplation of finitude and the cultivation of community, with its attendant goods and ends, I will address these two central components with a view to a bioethical framework. I will outline today's unique obstacles to an art of dying, and will conclude by identifying those areas that remain to be explored.

A Task for Bioethics?

As I argued in chapter 1, bioethics provides for medicine a common moral language and structure for resolving complex quandaries. The contributors to this volume have articulated means by which bioethics might, in limited ways, contribute to a contemporary *Ars moriendi*, but Lysaught in particular expresses grave reservations about the ability of bioethics to do so in any meaningfully substantive manner. I argue in response that a sufficiently robust conception of bioethics could indeed contribute to the establishment of a modern *Ars moriendi*.

Lysaught suggests that the methodology of bioethics is too limited to take on the project of articulating a contemporary art of dying. The best it can do, she says, is to "invent a generic and putatively neutral 'art of dying in hospitals' available to all patients," or to "call for medicine simply to make a space for individual patients to draw on rituals from their own traditions or invent rituals of their own making." Lysaught concludes, as does Callahan, that both of these options are insufficient. Instead, she proposes that bioethics consider the ethical framework of virtue ethics, an ethics that links practices with social ends; it is only within a virtue framework that the *Ars moriendi* can be grounded.

In fact, bioethics has seen in recent decades a revival of interest in a virtue-based approach to medical ethics. The physician and ethicist Edmund Pellegrino is well known for his systematic defense of virtue ethics and its application to the practice of medicine.[1] Additionally, other bioethicists operating under principle- or duty-based paradigms have taken on the virtues within their own frameworks.[2]

If such work has already been done, then why does Lysaught insist that bioethics has yet to incorporate virtue into its methodology? A complete answer is beyond the scope of this chapter, but briefly, I would suggest that although a virtue-based approach to bioethics has repeatedly been proposed, it hasn't yet become a dominant model for solving ethical problems in medicine. Neither has it featured prominently in how bioethics attends to dying and death. Some scholars find virtue ethics too complex for seamless application to bioethics, while others contend that it cannot reasonably address all the problems posed by bioethics.[3] Some argue that a virtue-based approach merely supplements other paradigms, and need not exist independently.[4]

And yet, since virtue ethics and bioethics do often overlap, Lysaught's proposal is perhaps not as impossible as it might seem. She suggests that for bioethics to create a framework for a modern *Ars moriendi*, it must do the following:

• incorporate properly a virtue methodology into its conventional methodology

• learn how to facilitate substantive clinical and cultural conversations about goods and ends

• ask serious questions of economics, attending to the myriad and powerful ways in which contemporary economic systems and philosophies quietly and often invisibly shape the patient, the clinical infrastructure, and biotechnology

• return dying to its proper, non-medical location, namely, the home or at least the local community

• make clear that practices at the deathbed must necessarily be related to a broader set of tradition-specific practices cultivated throughout life in the home, the congregation, and the community.

In other words, Lysaught is suggesting that in order for bioethics to be able to articulate a contemporary *Ars moriendi*, it must expand its methodology, generate substantive dialogue that challenges its own preconceptions, support efforts that expand home- or community-based dying, and support the role of specific communities in preparing their members for death.

Bioethics can surely rise to the challenges posed by the first four of these five tasks. However, one wonders whether it must falter at the fifth—which Lysaught associates with the Scottish philosopher Alasdair MacIntyre. Can bioethics create what she describes as community-specific and tradition-specific lifelong practices that are carried out by community members for and with the healthy as well as the dying, with the aim of shaping community members to die well? It is not clear whether bioethics on its own can achieve this; nor is it self-evident that bioethics has to go to this extreme in order to support an art of dying. But bioethics certainly can encourage individual communities to cultivate such practices; at the very least, it shouldn't get in the way of attempts by communities to do so.

Furthermore, it is worth bearing in mind that for more than half a millennium the practices of the *Ars moriendi* adapted organically to various religions, cultures, societies, ethnic groups, and countries without any interference or direction by bioethicists. Rather, individual communities recognized that the model offered by the *Ars moriendi* contained rich content that could be adapted in accordance with the determined ends, goods, and needs of their own communities.

Yet Lysaught insists that if bioethics doesn't create a MacIntyrean art of dying, "a good death will remain extraordinarily difficult to accomplish in the clinical context." And so she offers a second-tier approach to a good death, or to "a less medically malformed dying process." According to this approach, bioethics must seek to do the following:

• make the dying the principal directors of their own dying processes
• ensure that the dying know that they are dying
• enable the dying to take stock of their life, to express gratitude for life's goods as well as sorrow for its closure
• integrate practices of reconciliation, or "mutual forgiveness" among patients, family members, friends, and health care practitioners
• incorporate patients' communities integrally into the dying process
• acknowledge and attend to the wounds inflicted by death on patients' communities.

The content of these bioethical approaches to dying well—either the first-tier or the second-tier model—is surely more substantive than either the "generic and putatively neutral 'art of dying in hospitals' available to all patients" or the do-it-yourself approach to dying rituals that Lysaught and Callahan describe.

Even though this second-tier art of dying might seem to fall within the purview of contemporary bioethics, Lysaught remains unsure whether it is possible within the constraints of modern medicine. Palliative care, for example, attempts to accomplish these second-tier tasks; yet Lysaught asks whether palliative care, to use Callahan's term, may be "deforming" dying in new ways (a point Curlin raises in chapter 4). Lysaught also asks whether bioethics can persuasively address questions of ends and goods, and notes that different roles within the health care setting (patient versus hospital administrator, for example), will tend to predispose their protagonists to conceptions of ends and goods that are starkly different and even at odds. Can bioethics help to identify those goods and ends that are worth pursuing? Surely the answer is in the affirmative: bioethics *can* facilitate a deeper understanding; but whether it *will* is difficult to predict. Certainly success will not be readily or easily achieved.

Lysaught's remaining doubts can, I believe, be addressed by bioethicists, philosophers, and theologians, together with physicians, as long as their conceptions of bioethics are robust enough to allow for the integration of virtue ethics. Her concern that new approaches to death will "deform" the dying process in new ways renders it all the more important that bioethicists continue to engage, deeply and tenaciously, with questions pertaining to dying and death. Recently, the sponsors for an end-of-life ethics lecture series at a well-regarded university pulled their funding, purportedly claiming that "there is nothing new with end-of-life issues." The concerns raised by Lysaught, along with the ongoing temptation to medicalize further all aspects of life and death, reveal just how critical it is to maintain a rigorous bioethical discourse.

Having argued that bioethics, generally and generously considered, has the capacity to articulate a contemporary *Ars moriendi*, I next turn to *content*. As stated above, the art of dying cannot develop without two central components: recognition of finitude and development of community. I will consider these in turn.

Three Levels of Finitude

The threat of death has always prompted both individuals and their wider communities to contemplate finitude; but only recently has there arisen a need to consider a medical-scientific finitude. Any art of dying for the twenty-first century thus requires the admission of finitude on three levels: societal, individual, and medical-scientific.

Societal Contemplation of Finitude

First, a societal recovery of an *Ars moriendi* requires widespread recognition and examination of death, along the lines noted in chapter 1, which considered the Bubonic Plague, the American Civil War, the advent of cardiopulmonary resuscitation and mechanical ventilation, the death and dying movement, and the AIDS crisis. Each of these historical moments provoked widespread discussion of human finitude, either because a substantial portion of the population died suddenly (as with the Plague, Civil War, and AIDS), or because much of the population was affected by new biomedical developments, whether technological (life support) or theoretical (death and dying movement). After the Plague, the Catholic Church initiated the conversation by introducing the *Ars moriendi* texts, and by the time of the Civil War, preparation for death was considered part of a good upbringing, regardless of religious affiliation.

Is it possible to reinvigorate today the contemplation of finitude at a societal level without pestilence or war, and without revolutionary technology? The most viable scenario is perhaps that of a widespread campaign, probably driven (in the United States at least) by a combination of federal and local governments. Other efforts to raise societal awareness—as with breast or colon cancer screening,[5] or AIDS prevention[6]—have indeed been effective, and have had long-lasting positive consequences on public health. Although it might be difficult to imagine the launching in the near future of a national "Death: Think About It" campaign, it is more than possible that the costs incurred by end-of-life hospital care will soon become so burdensome that the federal government will be prompted to push the question of *how* one wants to die—or even *should* die—to the forefront of public discourse. Economic constraints will force the government either to encourage citizens to ponder their finitude as a matter of civic duty, or to implement rationing systems in order to curb the use of life-sustaining technology in medically futile situations. It is not unimaginable that the government would call upon professional bioethicists for help in crafting such a campaign.

Individual Contemplation of Finitude

The second level at which we must grapple with finitude is at the level of the individual, and here we might best be served by thinking of finitude as having at least three types: future, present, and conditional. Most people acknowledge at some point a *future* finitude, characterized by the statement "I will die." Such finitude rarely disrupts or threatens daily life; it remains distant, even theoretical. Fewer, perhaps, recognize a *present* finitude—an acute awareness of life's limits. The phrase "I am dying" describes this type. Such people may have confronted profound illness or may even have brushed with death. Even fewer still acknowledge a *conditional* finitude. The conditional type depends upon the state of one's health and requires at least one prior admission of present finitude. It pertains to individuals who are continuously reassessing themselves in light of new limitations or even temporary improvements in the context of chronic, progressive, and ultimately fatal disease. Such finitude might be characterized by the statement "I would be dying if … ." It requires individuals to make sense of themselves as beings who are not yet dead. Selwyn approximates this type in chapter 10; the transformation of AIDS from an acute, lethal illness to a chronic disease challenged patients and their caregivers to contemplate conditional finitude: "how to age with (as opposed to how to die with) the disease."

Note here that I am not proposing that these three types of individual finitude necessarily coexist. Though it is highly likely that for many patients death is at first hardly a reality (at best, a distant *future* finitude), and then becomes an increasing reality (approaching *present* finitude), I am less convinced that patients universally ponder their *conditional* finitude; how can one reassess oneself in light of new impairments or improvements if one has never first acknowledged a present finitude? These categories are meant to be descriptive and not proscriptive.

My patient Diana illustrates these different types of individual finitude. Before she became sick, she rarely contemplated her future finitude; busy and high-powered, she immersed herself fully in her present reality. Although her religious background did create some space for a general acknowledgment of mortality, this was for her, if anything, a distant future finitude. But, as Harrington and Sulmasy note in chapter 6, it is insufficient to hold, with Heidegger, that death is "an indeterminate something which first has to show up from somewhere, but right now is *not yet present* for oneself, and is thus no threat."[7] Death always delivers on mortality, whether one acknowledges that reality or not. After six months of illness, at about the time of our first meeting, Diana confronted death.

My second meeting with Diana was considerably calmer than my first. She had found the wherewithal in the interim to reflect on what it had been like to come face-to-face with her present finitude. She had come to the conclusion that during our first visit, she had been experiencing something of a catharsis. The shift from future to present finitude caused a thorough rearrangement of her inner life. Squarely facing her mortality compelled her to take stock of all she valued and to reorder her life in order to maximize remaining time and energy, doing what she loved, together with those she loved. According to the terms described by Latham in chapter 3, she began to seek after higher values while not dismissing strong values. Death's urgency began to lose its sway. A cathartic reordering of her life had fortified her against death.

But she wasn't dead. In fact, she was still quite alive and not worse than when I first met her. She couldn't walk long distances, and she required regular infusions of chemotherapy, a personal pharmacy of medications, and oxygen 24 hours of each day, but after nine months of illness she was probably even doing slightly better than when we first met. While the prospect of improvement was of course encouraging, it was also perplexing for both of us. According to her specialists' earlier advice, she should no longer be alive. Tempted as she was to pick up projects she had passed off to others and to rejoin committees from which she had resigned, Diana nevertheless remained conscious of death's shadow, of her present finitude, while attempting to make sense of her new limitations, her conditional finitude. I will never forget her words at our third meeting, which, I think, aptly characterize conditional finitude: "It's not the dying that's difficult; it's the trying to live."

The authors represented in this book have repeatedly pointed to the concepts of humility and vulnerability in the face of death. In Bishop's words, "What is needed, then, for existential meaning and purpose is not a better understanding of *how we die*. ... Nor is it better mastery of the dying body, as is suggested by medicine's never-ending quest to sustain human life. What is needed in the face of finitude is a kind of humility before that which must remain enigmatic for us mortals." Although humility might commonly be understood to imply meekness or low self-esteem, a better definition, and perhaps one which accords with virtue ethics, might be "having a clear perspective, and therefore respect, for one's place in context."[8] Recognition of finitude, then, *is* humility; it is the acknowledgment of and respect for the finite nature of one's existence. Humility goes hand-in-hand with vulnerability, or (literally) the possibility of being wounded. The blow of death inflicts a wound on life that is ultimately fatal. Once Diana had arrived at her present finitude, she never returned to a future finitude, but rather oscillated back and forth between a present and conditional finitude. Throughout she retained a clear perspective and healthy respect for her mortality, acknowledging all the while her susceptibility to the ultimate wounding.

Medical-Scientific Contemplation of Finitude

The third level at which finitude demands recognition, if there is to be any reinvigoration of the *Ars moriendi*, is at the level of scientists and physicians. Medical science and its practitioners are, as Bishop relays in chapter 2, necessarily fallible.[9] Knowledge itself admits of finitude. Bishop's vivid description of the untimely death of a young mother owing to misdiagnosis underscores the finitude of medical-scientific knowledge. But such finitude is hard to accept given the Babelic achievements of biomedicine over the last century: a near doubling of expected lifespan, development of life-saving antibiotics and chemotherapies, and successful transplantation of organs. For many, it seems unfathomable that medical science could face limitations.

Physicians in particular have a moral responsibility to be clear with their patients about medicine's limits, and bioethicists would do a service both to physicians and to patients by underscoring this fact. As leaders of medical teams and translators of medical science, doctors have unique responsibilities to patients—responsibilities they have because of their lengthy and highly technical training. I have been the primary care doctor for several patients with widely metastatic cancer, for example, whose oncologists never directly informed them that medicine had nothing left to offer and that they were dying. I recall two middle-aged women, both relatively new to me, and both diagnosed with widespread cancer refractory to treatment, who were completely unaware, until I told them, that they were nearing the "end of life." Neither had heard of advance directives, palliative care, or hospice. This is not an indictment of oncologists alone; such stories pervade all branches of medicine. No doubt their doctors had the best possible intentions despite not being forthright about their prognoses; indeed, instilling hope in the face of death is a difficult task. But avoiding direct conversation about the immediacy of death doesn't help patients to anticipate or prepare for death. If the doctor knows that a patient is dying and doesn't inform the patient, how can she make sense of herself, her remaining time, her relationships, her purpose? Even if bioethics can't deliver on the MacIntyrean model for dying, doctors shouldn't prevent their patients from immersing themselves in communities that have supported them throughout their lives, and could continue to support them in their dying.

Doctors, by virtue of their role as healers, want to cure their patients, but I would suggest that doctors should take a much more robust view of healing that includes, but is not limited to, curing. If medical science has no further treatments for a dying patient, the physician can pave the way toward the possibility of flourishing even in the face of death through a clear communication of medical-scientific finitude which leads in turn to the subject of the patient's finitude. Both Lantos and Callahan suggest a guiding principle, which Callahan articulates clearly: Patients shouldn't be forced to live longer than they might have lived in a pre-technological era. And Curlin underscores that hospice and palliative medicine—when practiced within the context of the goals of medicine—can instead help to achieve a recognition of finitude and an art of dying. It is recognition of finitude that helps bring into relief that which we most value. My patients who are cognizant of their dying are able to throw themselves into mending and strengthening relationships, cultivating memories with those who will survive them, putting their spiritual houses in order, and attending to the business aspects of life and death, such as dispensing with unneeded possessions and writing their wills. All of these activities lead to flourishing and a kind of beauty in the face of death; none of these activities may be achieved if the doctor doesn't make it clear that the patient is near death.

Three Levels of Community

Community, like finitude, helps us to make sense of what we most value—our goods and our ends—especially as our grasp loosens on the world around us. Community clarifies our sense of self, upholds us in our weakness, and facilitates the achievement of an art of dying. Indeed, I am aware of no proposal for a good death that *excludes* the role of community. In seeking to define a bioethical framework for a contemporary art of dying, no one expects that bioethics should provide that community. But, building from Lysaught's analysis, bioethics might facilitate substantive conversations about the integration of the dying person's community, practices, ends, and goods. I suggest here that community, like finitude, exists on three levels: familial, societal, and biomedical.

Familial Community

All of us stand to benefit from close relationships with friends or family members, in whose presence we can rest and unwind. This is even truer when we are sick. Just as women in childbirth don't typically invite their broader communities into the birthing chamber until the baby has appeared and the room has been cleaned, so too most dying patients share the messiness of death with only a select few. Often these intimate relationships are with those related by birth or marriage, but they can, of course, include relationships that might best be labeled "familial" even if no formal or genetic association exists. Latham tells the story of Mrs. M, who, while dying in the presence of her children, graciously handled an enthusiastic "get well" phone call from an acquaintance. Mrs. M felt no need to inform the caller that she was in her last hours of life; some information is worth sharing only within our closest community.

For Diana, her husband John provided just such a relationship, and during our second appointment, she brought him into the room so that we could meet. Even though the months accompanying his wife on her decline had for him been disconcerting, he was committed to seeing her through her illness and all the ugliness associated with it. Callahan's doubts expressed in chapter 9, about the typical seriousness of the vow to care for one another "in sickness and in health" are not borne out in this instance; John had no intention of offering anything less than his full support. In fact, John provided precisely the type of community that facilitates some of the charges spelled out by Lysaught. He could help Diana become the principal director of her dying process, could assist her in taking stock of her life and their life together, could aid her in the expression of gratitude for the goods of life as well as sorrow for its closure, could initiate practices of reconciliation and mutual forgiveness, and could attend to the wounds inflicted by death. John could even support deathbed practices related to the broader set of traditions cultivated by Diana throughout her life.

Not everyone recognizes this need for "familial community," even at the end of life. Yet the contributors to this book would uniformly view a lonely death as a failure of the *Ars moriendi*. Harrington and Sulmasy's account of the death of Susan Sontag illustrates clearly the nature of a death that lacks close community. They write:

Upon learning that her bone marrow transplant had failed, she screamed at the medical staff, at members of her family, and presumably at the universe itself, "But this means I'm going to die!" She went on to seek and receive further experimental chemotherapy, which also failed. She spent her last weeks in a state that a psychiatrist called "protective isolation," almost unable to express herself. She kept taking the chemotherapy pills until she could no longer swallow them, then died in a hospital bed, wasted, delirious, septic, and in shock.

Even if, as Sontag's son suggested, she had died a death that was "authentically hers" (by which he means that she went to the grave fighting for human progress), many would agree that such a death was less than "good" because Sontag ultimately failed to achieve in her dying the "high" values that Latham describes. In a state of "protective isolation" she could neither celebrate the successes of human progress nor permit her "community of care" to supplement her declining capacities (see Ridenour and Cahill, chapter 7). She didn't cultivate an *Ars moriendi*.

I would venture that such dying represents an extreme form of autonomy. What is needed instead, Ridenour and Cahill argue, is the retrieval of a Kantian understanding of autonomy. They begin by turning to Augustine, Aquinas, and Barth to make the case that human beings are by definition beings in relationship—"in a context of embedded vertical and horizontal community relations." They go on to assert that Kant's notion of autonomy "includes an implicit communal dimension … that treats all people as ends." Kantian autonomy is best understood not as libertarian, but as "moral agency directed by universal laws that serve a community of shared ends." Such a view of autonomy is implicitly relational.

Bioethics clearly cannot fabricate intimate relationships; however, by drawing on the work of philosophers and theologians, bioethicists can certainly make a case for, and support, the cultivation of intimate community—community that facilitates the achieving of high values even in death. And family members at the bedside can be empowered to carry out the tasks of an *Ars moriendi*. But, as Callahan describes, the burden on a solitary caretaker at the bedside can be enormous; for this reason, an art of dying requires the assistance of an even wider community.

Societal Community

For more than 500 years the *Ars moriendi* was practiced and experienced within the context of community; as Lantos puts it in chapter 8, "dying is a community affair." According to Ridenour and Cahill, "the human reality of death brings with it basic human needs, threats of suffering, and moral responsibilities that are shared across traditions and that require a communal response of 'accompanying' the dying." They suggest that "all ethical treatments of dying"—both spiritual and otherwise—should consider the basic human need for "'accompaniment' in the face of death."

The authors represented in this book consider different aspects of that broader community, many of which are essential to the articulation of a contemporary *Ars moriendi*. In showing how our collective care for critically ill children and their parents reflects how a society values its most vulnerable members, Lantos demonstrates that any ethical art of dying must pay particular attention to them; Callahan echoes that sentiment in regard to the most aged. Ridenour and Cahill suggest that the local community redouble its efforts to provide care to the dying, neighbors and volunteers providing respite for caretakers and local communities offering counseling. Callahan further broadens the definition of community by calling for federal economic support for elder care, with provisions for part-time caretakers. In describing the role of spirituality in an art of dying, Harrington and Sulmasy argue, through a narrative account of the life of Francis of Assisi, that true freedom in dying stems from choosing how to live in such a way that one may die well. And religious communities can provide the content their members need in order to live such that they die well. Thus, community—broadly considered—addresses the spiritual as well as the secular, and the political as well as the personal; taken together, these aspects of community can help to facilitate a contemporary art of dying.

My patient Diana had a vibrant community. Multi-generational and multi-disciplinary, it included colleagues from work and from professional organizations, fellow bird watchers, and members of her church. As she became ill, her broader community came to include those whom she called upon to assist her in her home. Diana had always been an extraordinary multitasker, and she excelled at cultivating deep and diverse relationships. From our first meeting, I had no doubt that her community would prove a source of strength even as she became increasingly debilitated. And as I cared for her over time, I witnessed firsthand just how integral her community was to her flourishing.

Biomedical Community

Intentionally or not, doctors often find themselves mulling over the concerns of their patients long after a clinic session has ended. Furthermore, some practice environments, such as small towns or close-knit university communities, lend themselves to doctors' and patients' seeing one another regularly. Certain other contexts also create opportunities for clinicians and patients to form tight communities—for example, Selwyn notes that during the early years of the AIDS crisis physicians viewed their patients as allies and attended their funerals, while broader society, in fear and ignorance, shunned both the doctors and the patients. In such contexts, it might not be surprising for physicians to consider patients as members of their broader community. My patient Diana was much on my mind as I composed this chapter, and I was amused to receive a note from her late one night while I was writing this section. I replied, told her what I had been writing, and asked "To what extent do patients view doctors as part of their broader community?"

It is undoubtedly fair to say that many patients do view members of their health care team as members of their broader community, especially within the context of a long-standing doctor-patient relationship or of acute decline of a patient with a chronic illness. The medical-team model has done much to add to the number of patients who hold this view; even if a patient doesn't care for his or her physician's bedside manner, the patient's relationships with other members of a medical team, such as a social worker or a mid-level provider, may offer the emotional connections the patient needs. In chapter 7, Ridenour and Cahill tell the story of the bioethicist Marilyn Martone's experience in the hospital as her daughter faced death. Martone recounts the importance of "practicing community" with other patients' families, medical professionals, and hospital staff. For Martone, that tangible solidarity within the hospital seemed as important as the community offered by friends and family members.

The momentum within medical practice is toward accomplishing a task. As Jeffrey Bishop writes in *The Anticipatory Corpse*, "medicine is about doing and not about thinking."[10] But bioethicists can help members of a medical team to *think* about how they can serve dying patients better. Bioethics can help physicians recognize that they can provide more than pain relief and technical management of death. Doctors may assist their patients in achieving an art of dying by encouraging them to take stock of their lives, to integrate practices of reconciliation, and to acknowledge the wounds of death.

Obstacles to a Contemporary Art of Dying

In addition to the bioethical constraints described above, other obstacles to a contemporary *Ars moriendi* will persist.

First, there will always be people who lack the willingness to confront finitude, whether because of deeply held beliefs (as in the case of Susan Sontag) or because of fear, ignorance, discomfort, or inability to comprehend the incomprehensible. Bishop, drawing on Hegel, suggests in chapter 2 that it is impossible to think of death in the first person, since "death is a concept for which we have no image or representation." Yet human beings possess the ability to reason about what is at present unfamiliar, even without knowing, for example, precisely what death entails. Indeed, this sort of anticipation characterizes much of life, as when a child thinks of kindergarten without a concrete representation or when an expectant mother anticipates the birth of her own baby. The child has heard about school and the expectant mother has seen newborns, but they don't know for themselves what the experiences will be like.

Second, even among those who admit of life's limits, there will continue to be many who nevertheless become incapacitated once the subject of death actually presents itself. It is especially problematic when doctors are unable to handle death. Selwyn juxtaposes his early years as an AIDS doctor—when death was "not a stranger to anyone"—with the "newer generations of AIDS care providers" who "often don't dwell on end-of-life care or the anticipation of death" but rather "pay more attention to treating the acute complications and monitoring the exacerbations and remissions of a slowly progressive illness." Selwyn notes that this inhibits a doctor's ability to "accompany patients through these phases when they do occur, as they inevitably do for all of us."

Third, community at all three levels described (familial, societal, and biomedical) will be difficult for many to achieve. Fragmentation of societal and familial relationships is nothing new, but globalization, increased mobility, and the shift to electronically maintained relationships probably will weaken the foundations of community still further. Medicine's increasing experimentation with virtual office visits ("e-visits") also challenges the integrity of the medical profession's contribution to community. As has been emphasized repeatedly, an *Ars moriendi* is not possible without a strong community.

Fourth, to the extent that physicians are relied upon for guidance in an art of dying, time pressures will hinder effective communication. After my first visit with Diana, which pushed me hopelessly behind schedule, I scheduled her next two visits at my customary lunch break in order to ensure that we would have enough time to address her existential ponderings. But by our sixth visit, she was nestled into my schedule in a standard "return patient" slot, surrounded by 26 others. I remember thinking how much deeper our conversations had been at our first few appointments. Though I didn't sense that I was conveniently ignoring a need on the day of that sixth visit, I regretted that I couldn't simply "be present," as Selwyn was with his patients in the early years of the AIDS crisis. Selwyn notes that as treatments became more effective, care of patients with AIDS became more reductionist. Whereas in the early days of AIDS "it felt as if the doctor and the patient were allied against the disease," he writes, "it now sometimes feels as if the doctor and the therapy are allied against the patient." The obstacle of time encourages a reductionist approach to medicine, and reductionist approaches don't foster an art of dying.

One of the most powerful features of the *Ars moriendi* was its incorporation into the routines of daily life. This leads to a fifth challenge: daily discipline. In the absence of the ravages of plague or war, the only way to cultivate the practices of an art of dying is through personal and community-wide discipline. But daily discipline may not have the cultural purchase that it once did. In the clinic I attempt to initiate such conversations by taking my end-of-life discussions with patients beyond simple questions of advance directives. In the community I have taken these concerns to my congregation, and its leaders have begun to talk openly and actively about an art of dying well and its relationship to the art of living well. Beyond such efforts and my own commitment to speaking openly about death, the incorporation of an *Ars moriendi* into daily life remains elusive.

Further Work

The demands of a project to frame a contemporary art of dying seem limitless. The more I read and write and speak on this subject, the more questions present themselves for analysis. I will conclude by mentioning two concrete areas that deserve further attention.

First, it is worth questioning the extent to which the cultural shift from viewing illness and death as inevitable to seeing them as aberrations affects the possibility of a retrieval of the *Ars moriendi*. Selwyn describes the problem in the context of caring for patients with AIDS, but he offers no solution: "Before treatment existed, when death was inevitable and the trajectory was swift and uniform, it seemed almost that dying was a matter of 'fate'—that is, something unavoidable, universal, and expected. Once effective disease-modifying treatments became available, 'fate' was somehow transformed into 'tragedy,' a separation between what was happening and what might have been, a terrain of 'what ifs,' choices taken and not taken, and more a function of individual responsibility and agency." But society, doctors, and patients don't merely view illness as a deviation from normal; aging itself has become problematic. Not long ago, when I was the primary care doctor on call for a group of internists, a young medical trainee paged me from the emergency room. He just wanted me to know, he said, that one of my colleague's "very high risk" patients was being discharged from the emergency room because the medical work-up hadn't revealed a cause for his now-resolved 20-minute dizzy spell. I asked "What makes the patient 'high risk'?" "Well," the trainee replied, "he doesn't have any medical problems, but he is 95." If, in addition to illness, aging itself has become an aberration, how will this affect the recovery of an art of dying?

Also to be explored is the possibility of a retrieval of the *Ars moriendi* in an era in which the demographics of living and dying differ so markedly from those that obtained during the half-millennium when the *Ars moriendi* was at its peak. Until the twentieth century, people lived shorter lives, and the intervals between birth, witnessing the death of others, and one's own death were much shorter. It is no wonder then that young healthy people would contemplate their finitude and prepare for death. But we age differently today. My 70-year-old patients often claim that they don't "feel their age"—that is, they feel younger than they had expected to feel at 70. Since they fail to recognize their own aging, and since medicine excels at delaying death, it remains to be investigated how the substance of a contemporary *Ars moriendi* will continue to change as the needs of successive dying generations change.

Grounded in bioethics, this book seeks to articulate a preliminary theoretical framework for an art of dying in the twenty-first century. After nearly four years of concerted effort, we are conscious that the work isn't complete. Rather than delay completion of the book, I choose to recognize the finitude of the project; out of respect for the community of contributing writers, I bring the book to a timely end.

But the larger project continues, much like the experiences of those, like Diana, who have provided impetus to the process. I opened this chapter with her story because I continue to be amazed at how clearly and consistently she lives out the substance of the *Ars moriendi*. The art of her dying seems to reflect the fullness of the art of her living. And she is actively structuring her days such that she is flourishing even in her dying.

Notes

1. Edmund D. Pellegrino, "The Virtuous Physician and the Ethics of Medicine," in *Virtue and Medicine: Explorations in the Character of Medicine*, ed. Earl Shelp (Reidel, 1985). See also Edmund D. Pellegrino and David C. Thomasma, *The Virtues in Medical Practice* (Oxford University Press, 1993).

2. See, for example, Tom L. Beauchamp and James F. Childress, *Principles of Biomedical Ethics*, fourth edition (Oxford University Press, 1994).

3. Stephen Holland, "The Virtue Ethics Approach to Bioethics," *Bioethics* 25 (2011): 192–201; Karen M. Meagher, "Considering Virtue: Public Health and Clinical Ethics," *Journal of Evaluation in Clinical Practice* 17 (2011): 888–893.

4. Lynn A. Jansen, "The Virtues in Their Place: Virtue Ethics in Medicine," *Theoretical Medicine* 21 (2000): 263–264.

5. Jeanette Kamell Mitchell and Kieron S. Leslie, "Melanoma Death Prevention: Moving Away From the Sun," *Journal of the American Academy of Dermatology* 68 (2013): 169–175.

6. Wayne D. Johnson et al., "Behavioral Interventions to Reduce Risk for Sexual Transmission of HIV Among Men Who Have Sex with Men," *Cochrane Database Systematic Review* 3 (2008): CD001230.

7. Martin Heidegger, *Being and Time*, tr. Joan Stambaugh (State University of New York Press, 2010), 243.

8. "Humility," Wikipedia (http://en.wikipedia.org/wiki/Humility).

9. In chapter 2, note especially Bishop's description of Gorovitz and MacIntyre's "necessary fallibility" as a statement about the finitude of knowledge.

10. Jeffrey P. Bishop, *The Anticipatory Corpse: Medicine, Power, and the Care of the Dying* (University of Notre Dame Press, 2011), 21.

Contributors

Jeffrey P. Bishop, MD, PhD is a social and moral philosopher teaching medical ethics and philosophy at Saint Louis University. He is also a physician. He holds the Tenet Endowed Chair in Health Care Ethics and is Director of the Albert Gnaegi Center for Health Care Ethics. He is the author of *The Anticipatory Corpse: Medicine, Power, and the Care of the Dying* (2011).

Lisa Sowle Cahill, PhD is the J. Donald Monan, S.J., Professor of Theology at Boston College. A past president of the Catholic Theological Society of America (1992–93) and of the Society of Christian Ethics (1997–98), she is a member of the American Academy of Arts and Sciences. Her publications include *Theological Bioethics: Participation, Justice, and Change* (2005) and *Global Justice, Christology and Christian Ethics* (2013).

Daniel Callahan, PhD is Senior Research Scholar and President Emeritus of the Hastings Center. A co-founder of the Hastings Center in 1969, he served as its president from 1969 until 1996. He is also a co-director of the Yale-Hastings Program in Ethics and Health Policy. An elected member of the Institute of Medicine and National Academy of Sciences, he is the author or editor of more than 41 books, including *In Search of the Good: A Life in Bioethics* (2012) and *The Roots of Bioethics: Health, Progress, Technology, Death* (2012).

Farr A. Curlin, MD is a hospice and palliative care physician. A founder and a former co-director of the Program on Medicine and Religion at the University of Chicago, he is now the Josiah C. Trent Professor of Medical Humanities at Duke University, working with colleagues in the medical school and in the Duke Divinity School to foster scholarship, study, and training at the intersection of medicine, ethics, and religion.

Lydia S. Dugdale, MD is an assistant professor of medicine and the Associate Director for the Program on Biomedical Ethics at Yale School of Medicine. A graduate of the University of Chicago's Pritzker School of Medicine, she is currently a Faculty Scholar in the Program on Medicine and Religion at the University of Chicago, with funding from the John Templeton Foundation. As part of the Templeton award, she is studying part-time at the Yale Divinity School, where she is pursuing an MA degree in ethics.

Michelle Harrington, AM is a doctoral candidate in Constructive Studies in Religious Ethics at the University of Chicago Divinity School. Her dissertation is titled Laying Down One's Life: Autonomy in the Time of Medicalized Death. After receiving a BA in social and political ethics from Oglethorpe University, she was appointed a dissertation junior fellow for the 2012–13 academic year at the Martin Marty Center for the Advanced Study of Religion at the University of Chicago Divinity School. She is also a graduate of the MacLean Center for Clinical Medical Ethics.

John Lantos, MD is Director of the Children's Mercy Hospital Bioethics Center in Kansas City. A leader in the field of bioethics for thirty years, he was a resident at Children's National Medical Center in Washington during the Baby Doe controversy, which kindled a life-long interest in tradeoffs between quality of life and survival. He has written or spoken on ethical issues in bone marrow transplantation for hemoglobinopathies, ECMO for respiratory failure, hypothermia for anoxic encephalopathy, and other innovative therapies. He has been president of the two leading bioethics organizations in the United States (the American Society for Bioethics and Humanities and the American Society of Law, Medicine and Ethics), has testified before the President's Council on Bioethics, has appeared on Oprah, and has been named one of the best pediatricians in the Midwest by *Ladies Home Journal*.

Stephen R. Latham, JD, PhD—formerly a health care business and regulatory attorney and Director of Ethics Standards for the American Medical Association—now serves as Director of Yale University's Interdisciplinary Center for Bioethics. A graduate of Harvard College, Harvard Law School, and the University of California at Berkeley, he was a graduate fellow at Harvard's Safra Center on Ethics and a research fellow at the University of Edinburgh's Institute for Advanced Studies in the

Humanities. He is a former member of Connecticut's Stem Cell Research Advisory Committee and of the board of the American Society for Bioethics and Humanities, which gave him its distinguished service award in 2010. He serves on the Pediatric Ethics Committee at Yale's Children's Hospital and chairs Yale's social science institutional review board. His publications on health law and ethics have appeared in numerous medical and bioethics journals, law reviews, and university press books. He is an associate editor of the forthcoming fourth edition of the *Encyclopedia of Bioethics* and a contributing editor of the *Hastings Center Report*.

M. Therese Lysaught, PhD is a professor of Catholic moral theology and health care ethics at the Institute of Pastoral Studies at Loyola University Chicago, with a secondary appointment in the Neiswanger Institute of Bioethics at Loyola's Stritch School of Medicine. She consults with health care systems on issues of mission, theology, and ethics. She has done research on the anointing of the sick, on genetics, on gene therapy, on human embryonic stem cell research, and on end-of-life issues. Currently she is involved with the Human Powered Nebulizer Project, with research funded by the Science of Virtue Program of the Arete Foundation at the University of Chicago examining the cultural constructions of virtue, vice, and poverty in contemporary work on the neurosciences. Her scholarly monograph *Anointing of the Sick and the Theo-Political Economy of Medicine* is expected to be published by 2016. In addition to authoring almost 50 articles and book chapters and presenting almost 100 invited lectures and conference papers, she has served as an advisor to the Catholic Health Association. She currently serves on the Board of Directors of the Society of Christian Ethics and on the editorial board of the *Journal of Moral Theology*.

Autumn Alcott Ridenour, PhD is Assistant Professor of Religious and Theological Studies at Merrimack College. She recently received a PhD in Theological Ethics from Boston College. Before attending Boston College, she received an MA degree in ethics from the Yale Divinity School and worked at Yale University's Interdisciplinary Center for Bioethics.

Peter A. Selwyn, MD, MPH is Professor of Family Medicine, Internal Medicine, and Epidemiology and Population Health and Chairman of the Department of Family and Social Medicine at Montefiore Medical Center and Albert Einstein College of Medicine in the Bronx. Director of Palliative Care Program at Montefiore Medical Center, he also directs Montefiore's

Office of Community Health. He holds degrees from Swarthmore College, Harvard Medical School, and Columbia University. As Medical Director of the Montefiore Substance Abuse Treatment Program, he was involved in some of the earliest studies of AIDS and substance abuse, developing model programs to provide care for high-risk populations in the Bronx. A former Associate Director of the AIDS Program at the Yale School of Medicine, he has been Medical Director of Leeway, Inc. (a 40-bed AIDS-dedicated skilled nursing facility in New Haven) since 1995. He has published more than 170 articles, book chapters, monographs, and reviews on HIV/AIDS, substance abuse, palliative care, underserved populations, primary care, and health disparities. He is a co-editor of the US Health Resources and Services Administration's Clinical Guide to Supportive and Palliative Care for HIV/ AIDS (2003) and the author of *Surviving the Fall: The Personal Journey of an AIDS Doctor* (2000), which was nominated for the National Book Award.

Daniel Sulmasy, MD, PhD is the Kilbride-Clinton Professor of Medicine and Ethics in the Department of Medicine and Divinity School at the University of Chicago, where he also serves as Associate Director of the MacLean Center for Clinical Medical Ethics. He has previously held faculty positions at New York Medical College and at Georgetown University. He received AB and MD degrees from Cornell University, completed his residency, chief residency, and post-doctoral fellowship in General Internal Medicine at the Johns Hopkins Hospital, then received a PhD in philosophy from Georgetown University in 1995. He has served on numerous governmental advisory committees, and was appointed to the Presidential Commission for the Study of Bioethical Issues by President Obama in April of 2010. His research interests encompass both theoretical and empirical investigations of the ethics of end-of-life decision making, ethics education, and spirituality in medicine. He has authored or edited five books: *The Healer's Calling* (1997), *Methods in Medical Ethics* (first edition 2001, second edition 2010), *The Rebirth of the Clinic* (2006), *A Balm for Gilead* (2006), and *Safe Passage: A Global Spiritual Sourcebook for Care at the End of Life* (2014). He also serves as editor-in-chief of the journal *Theoretical Medicine and Bioethics*.

Michael L. Gross, *Bioethics and Armed Conflict: Moral Dilemmas of Medicine and War*

Karen F. Greif and Jon F. Merz, *Current Controversies in the Biological Sciences: Case Studies of Policy Challenges from New Technologies*

Deborah Blizzard, *Looking Within: A Sociocultural Examination of Fetoscopy*

Ronald Cole-Turner, editor, *Design and Destiny: Jewish and Christian Perspectives on Human Germline Modification*

Holly Fernandez Lynch, *Conflicts of Conscience in Health Care: An Institutional Compromise*

Mark A. Bedau and Emily C. Parke, editors, *The Ethics of Protocells: Moral and Social Implications of Creating Life in the Laboratory*

Jonathan D. Moreno and Sam Berger, editors, *Progress in Bioethics: Science, Policy, and Politics*

Eric Racine, *Pragmatic Neuroethics: Improving Understanding and Treatment of the Mind-Brain*

Martha J. Farah, editor, *Neuroethics: An Introduction with Readings*

Jeremy R. Garrett, editor, *The Ethics of Animal Research: Exploring the Controversy*

Books Acquired under the Editorship of Arthur Caplan

Sheila Jasanoff, editor, *Reframing Rights: Bioconstitutionalism in the Genetic Age*

Christine Overall, *Why Have Children? The Ethical Debate*

Yechiel Michael Barilan, *Human Dignity, Human Rights, and Responsibility: The New Language of Global Bioethics and Bio-Law*

Tom Koch, *Thieves of Virtue: When Bioethics Stole Medicine*

Timothy F. Murphy, *Ethics, Sexual Orientation, and Choices about Children*

Daniel Callahan, *In Search of the Good: A Life in Bioethics*

Robert Blank, *Intervention in the Brain: Politics, Policy, and Ethics*

Gregory E. Kaebnick and Thomas H. Murray, editors, *Synthetic Biology and Morality: Artificial Life and the Bounds of Nature*

Dominic A. Sisti, Arthur L. Caplan, and Hila Rimon-Greenspan, editors, *Applied Ethics in Mental Healthcare: An Interdisciplinary Reader*

Barbara K. Redman, *Research Misconduct Policy in Biomedicine: Beyond the Bad-Apple Approach*

Russell Blackford, *Humanity Enhanced: Genetic Choice and the Challenge for Liberal Democracies*

Nicholas Agar, *Truly Human Enhancement: A Philosophical Defense of Limits*

Bruno Perreau, *The Politics of Adoption: Gender and the Making of French Citizenship*

Carl Schneider, *The Censor's Hand: The Misregulation of Human-Subject Research*

Lydia S. Dugdale, editor, *Dying in the Twenty-First Century: Toward a New Ethical Framework for the Art of Dying Well*

Index

Printed in the United States
By Bookmasters